PRIMARY CARE OTOLARYNGOLOGY

American Academy of Otolaryngology—
Head and Neck Surgery Foundation

Editor: Mark K. Wax, MD

J. Gregory Staffel, MD

James C. Denneny III, MD

David E. Eibling, MD

Jonas T. Johnson, MD

Margaret A. Kenna, MD

Karen T. Pitman, MD

Clark A. Rosen, MD

Scott W. Thompson, MD

And Members of the Core Otolaryngology Education Faculty
American Academy of Otolaryngology—
Head and Neck Surgery Foundation

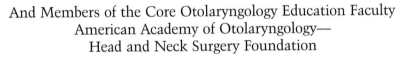

Dr. Gregory Staffel first authored this short introduction to otolaryngology for medical students at the University of Texas School for the Health Sciences in San Antonio in 1996. Written in conversational style, peppered with hints for learning (such as "read an hour a day"), and short enough to digest in one or two evenings, the book was a "hit" with medical students.

Dr. Staffel graciously donated his book to the American Academy of Otolaryngology—Head and Neck Surgery Foundation to be used as a basis for this primer. It has been revised, edited and is now in the second printing. This edition has undergone an extensive review, revision and updating. We believe that you, the reader, will find this book enjoyable and informative. We anticipate that it will whet your appetite for further learning in the discipline that we love and have found most intriguing. It should start your journey into otolaryngology, the field of Head and Neck Surgery.

Enjoy!

Mark K. Wax, MD

Editor: Primary Care Otolaryngology
Chair: Core Otolaryngology Education Faculty
American Academy of Otolaryngology—Head and Neck Surgery Foundation

Table of Contents

1. Introduction to Clinical Rotation 3

2. Keeping Track of Patients 7

3. Postoperative Fevers 11

4. ENT Emergencies 14

5. Otitis Media 23

6. Hearing Loss 33

7. Dizziness 40

8. Facial Nerve Paralysis 45

9. Rhinology, Nasal Obstruction and Sinusitis 49

10. How to Read a Sinus CT Scan 57

11. Maxillofacial Trauma 62

12. Facial Plastic Surgery 69

13. Salivary Gland Disease 75

14. Thyroid Cancer 79

15. Head and Neck Cancer 84

16. Skin Cancer 93

17. Pediatric Otolaryngology 97

Introduction to Clinical Rotation

The goals of this book are to make you a good clinician . . .

The goals of this book are to make you a good **clinician** and to teach you basic **Ear**, **Nose**, and **Throat (ENT) medicine and surgery**.

Sometimes individuals have trouble transitioning from being a 2nd-year medical student, where they are truly a student, to becoming a health care professional, which is that metamorphosis that occurs in the 3rd and 4th year of medical school. This involves learning to carry yourself and act as a health care professional.

The process starts with the student's appearance (clothing and grooming), punctuality, composure, **acceptance of responsibility**, and **interactions with patients and other health care team members**. You need to really listen to patients. It's helpful for students to be carefully observant of their professors in important but unnoticed activities such as their demeanor, comments, and interaction with house staff and patients. Students learn a lot through observing care of patients.

It is difficult to understand medical students' role in the health care team. Become an active member of the health care team. Interns, residents, and attendings are overworked and spread quite thin. However, medical students frequently have extra time to spend with their patients, talking to the patients about their **past medical problems, family, and social aspects** as they pertain to their disease process and, most important, truly establishing a **patient-doctor relationship**. This type of relationship establishes the medical student as an important part of the health care team, beneficial to the overall care provided to the patient. It also establishes long-term behaviors for that medical student, which translates into the development of an excellent future physician.

A few basic rules will help you to become a good clinician. During the 3rd year, you may have conflicting responsibilities, such as being at a lecture while needing to draw a patient's blood. In general, **the priority should be the care of the patient**.

If it is an important blood test and you can't get someone to do it for you, you may need to miss the lecture. These situations don't actually come up that often, and if patient care is your main goal over the long run, most people will see it.

There are two kinds of doctors: those who read and those who don't. Read about your patients. You should read textbooks because they cover the basics and 90% of people don't know what is in them. Articles are for later. It doesn't matter which textbook you read, because if the information is important, it will come up again and you will find it again in later reading. If the information is unimportant, it won't come up very often.

So now you have 4 patients and you go home. You got up at 5:00 a.m. to make it to rounds. You get home at 7:00 p.m. after your last postop note. After you have petted the dog and made supper, it's 8:30. You deserve a break, so you watch TV for an hour. You are ready to read, and you realize your patient has hypertension (HTN), chronic obstructive pulmonary disease (COPD), diabetes, and a pleomorphic adenoma. There's no way you can read about all that tonight, and you have to get up at 5:00 a.m. tomorrow. So it's in the hay, and the next morning you don't really know why we even treat asymptomatic hypertension in the first place. Solution: **Read for an hour every day.** Afterward you can do whatever you want and not feel guilty or overwhelmed. You will also be amazed at how well you do. Most students don't average anywhere near that.

Read about your patients. Remember Darwin's theory of medical education: "It can't be that rare if you are seeing it."

We know that you, as medical students, aspire to the highest ideals of professionalism. We know that you will always have a neat appearance and a pleasant personality. We know that you will do completely thorough histories and physicals (H&Ps). You will be very compassionate to all your patients and coworkers, and you will always be willing and ready to learn. It has been our experience that all students know this is expected of them. However, there is one important caveat that is often not addressed in medical education. It is as much your responsibility to know your limitations as it is to know about treating patients. If you are trying hard, reading an hour every day, and truly interested, then if you are asked a question to which you don't know the answer, it's

Don't let your schooling get in the way of your education.

Mark Twain

perfectly legitimate and indeed expected that you simply answer, "I don't know." Nobody knows everything.

If you use the information you already have, you will do surprisingly well if you guess at an answer. But if your answer is only a guess, qualify it by pointing out that you hadn't specifically known the answer. Integrity—an absolute commitment to honesty—is a prerequisite for becoming a physician.

Although you may not know that much quite yet in your clinical career, you do have one secret weapon as a student: enthusiasm. Residents are often tired and grouchy, as you probably have noticed, but having an enthusiastic student around makes a difference.

The 2nd goal of this book is to teach you a little about common ENT problems. Since the great majority of you won't be **otolaryngologists**, it becomes much more important for you to understand how to recognize potentially dangerous problems, which should be referred to an ENT doctor, as well as how to manage uncomplicated problems that don't require referral to an otolaryngologist.

5

It is astonishing with how little reading a doctor can practice medicine, but it is not astonishing how badly he may do it.

Sir William Osler

Questions, Section #1

1. Your highest professional priority throughout your 3rd year and the rest of your career should be _____.

2. One way to learn as much as possible, without feeling overwhelmed, during the 3rd year is to _____.

3. When faced with two conflicting responsibilities, _____ should always be your highest priority.

4. If you guess at a question on rounds, you should _____.

5. The key to a happy career in medicine is to make _____ your highest professional priority.

6. The key to happiness in medicine is to keep in mind question #5 and _____.

7. In all countries of the world, a common vein through medicine is to keep as the first priority _____.

8. The key to a well-balanced and happy medical school career is to _____.

Answers

1. THE CARE OF THE PATIENT
2. READ FOR AN HOUR EVERY DAY
3. THE CARE OF THE PATIENT
4. QUALIFY YOUR ANSWER
5. THE CARE OF THE PATIENT
6. READ FOR AN HOUR EVERY DAY
7. THE CARE OF THE PATIENT
8. READ FOR AN HOUR EVERY DAY

On the ENT service, most patients spend very little time in the hospital, and keeping track of everything about the patient isn't worth your time. However, certain key information is needed on each patient, and you should learn how to keep this information in a usable format. The general surgery patient and internal medicine patient are apt to be on the 2-week plan, and this system is offered to help you with your rounds duties. Perhaps most important, a list of patients and their diseases is an ideal way to review and pick topics for additional reading. (Remember, you are reading an hour every day.)

The system involves **3 x 5-inch note cards**, preferably blank (but if they have lines, it will do). You must write small, of course—if you want to write big, you should have been a 1st grade teacher or an attending. The basic idea is shown in Figure 2.1. A few pointers...

An alternative is to use a PDA with commercial Data Software. This system allows storage of the data, so should you wish to "retrieve" a memorable patient experience, it will be available.

Don't stamp the patient's name on your card. You waste valuable space soon to be used by the discreet doctor. Also, memorize a format such as the one below and you won't waste space labeling what goes where.

Name: SMITH, John   MR# 12-345-6785   Rm# 233A
64 yo WM w/tonsil Ca, CAD, HTN, DM

History

NKDA
Meds: start/stop date
cefazolin, metronidazole, 8/24.

Ba swallow 8/30, no extravasation.
Study: date,
      results

Urine 8/27, 100K/ml. *E. coli*
culture: date,
      results

Path: SCCa, margins, 8/22 LN +

Figure 2.1.

Leave space for the room number to change. It is also useful to put the floor and wing, unless you know for sure where the room is. On the back of the card, Figure 2.2, you will need room for a lot of data in a small space. I used to start a new column for each day, but I found I had space for only about 5 days' data, so I started using serial spacing. In that way, I could usually get about 7-10 days on 1 card. If the patient stays longer, you can tape another card to the original in such a way that they open like a book. I never needed more than 2 cards for a patient.

8/24	8/25			
POD 1: cefazolin/metronidazole	POD 2: cefazolin/metronidazole			
Tmax: 38.5	(etc....)			
i/o: 2700/1380				
JPs: A 170, B 125				
(Labs...)				

Figure 2.2.

What you'll notice if you look closely and understand the system is that you know everything about the patients during their whole stay. When the chief resident asks, "What was his creatinine 3 days ago?"—you know it!

Differential Diagnosis:

Every time you see a new patient, you begin to formulate a **differential diagnosis** for him or her. Most of us begin by doing this randomly, usually the **5 most recent diagnoses** we have **seen for this set of symptoms and physical findings**. This works when you have seen several thousand patients, but it's not as useful if you have seen only 100 or so. A useful trick is to use an acronym that represents a **system based on disease categories** (such as "Vitamin C," see below). Try it for yourself, and practice using it on all your patients. You'll find that it or another system will be a big help in organizing your thoughts when you're confused or during high-stress rounds.

Vitamin C

Vascular

Infectious

Traumatic

Autoimmune (or anatomic)

Metabolic

Iatrogenic or Idiopathic

Neoplastic

Congenital

Question, Section #2

1. Vitamin C is one way of organizing a differential diagnosis list.

    V_____,

    I_____,

    T_____,

    A_____,

    M_____,

    I_____,

    N_____,

    C_____.

Answer

1. VASCULAR
    INFECTIOUS
    TRAUMATIC
    AUTOIMMUNE
    METABOLIC
    IDIOPATHIC OR IATROGENIC
    NEOPLASTIC
    CONGENITAL

In surgery the differential diagnosis, as it relates to specific symptoms, depends on the time since the procedure has been completed. For example, if a person has a fever, the most likely cause is dictated somewhat by the **postoperative day (POD)**. Remembering the **five W's of postop fever—Wind, Water, Walking, Wound, and Wonder drugs**—as a useful memory tool when you are following patients after surgery.

POD 1-2: **Wind: Atelectasis (without air)** often causes a fever. Reasons include being on a ventilator, inadequate sighs during surgery, and (in the general surgery patient) incisional pain on deep breathing. This is treated with incentive **spirometry** because there is evidence that **deep inspiration** prevents atelectasis better than just coughing.

POD 3-5: **Water: Urinary tract infections (UTIs)** are common here. Foley catheters are sometimes still in place.

POD 4-6: **Walking: Deep venous thrombosis** can occur. This is more of a problem in patients undergoing pelvic, orthopedic, or general surgery than in head and neck surgery. Subcutaneous, low-dose **heparin** and **venous compression devices** reduce the incidence of **thromboembolization.** Walking the patient on POD 1 is the best way to prevent this complication.

11

POD 5-7: **Wound**: Most wound infections occur during this period. **Preoperative antibiotics** are important to prevent or reduce the risk of infection in head and neck surgery that crosses **mucosal linings**.

POD 7+: **Wonder drugs:** Drugs can cause fevers. (Note that in obstetrics and gynecology, this W is "Womb," and it precedes "Wonder drugs.")

How to Present on Rounds:

Patient presentations should be **goal directed**. Presentations should follow this format:

"Mr. Jones is a 63-year-old man with a **T3** cancer

of the tonsil that failed radiation. He initially presented with a 2-month history of pain and a **nonhealing ulcer** on the left tonsil. He underwent 6 weeks of radiotherapy and was disease free for 7 months. His tumor recurred, and three days ago, he underwent a mandibulotomy, neck dissection, hemiglosectomy and partial pharyngectomy with tracheostomy. A radial forearm free tissue transfer was the reconstruction. He is **afebrile** (this means less than 38.5), and his **perioperative antibiotics** have been discontinued. He is tolerating his tube feeds at 100 cc per hour, and his drains have each put out 30 cc over the last 24 hours."

The last sentence in your presentation should always start with "The plan is...." For example: "The plan is to remove the drains today, continue the tube feedings, and start feeding the patient by mouth at one week post surgery." We also plan to cap his **tracheostomy** tube and remove it if he tolerates having it plugged. We have contacted social work in order to make sure that he has a place to go when we are ready to discharge him at day 8 or 9 postop."

For a general surgery patient, the presentation may be something like this:

"This is day 1 post colon resection for Mrs. Jones, a 60-year-old woman with colon cancer found on endoscopy obtained because of a positive test for occult blood in the stool."

Discuss ins, outs, and drains. Finally, your last sentence should start with "The plan is...." Always think of what you need to do to send the patient home. For example, if she still isn't eating and needs **IVs** for fluid intake, the object would be to get her eating.

Questions, Section #3

1. The 5 W's of postoperative fever are _____, _____, _____,_____, and _____.

2. A fever on postoperative day 5-7 may be due to an infection of the _____.

3. A fever on the night of surgery is most likely due to _____.

Answers
1. WIND, WATER, WALKING, WOUND, WONDER DRUGS
2. WOUND
3. ATELECTASIS

14

Airway:

Airway emergencies are uncommon, but devastating when they do happen. Whether the patient lives or dies—or worse, lives for years in a coma—depends on the ability of those caring for him or her to **recognize, access, and manage** the airway. ENT physicians are experts in airway management, but often not nearby when needed. The advanced trauma life support (ATLS) course you probably have taken or will take emphasizes management of airway emergencies. Predicting when difficulty will occur and being able to manage the difficult airway without it becoming an emergency is an even more valuable skill. Later, this chapter will list 3 types of airway difficulties that you might encounter.

A good rule of thumb about a **tracheotomy** is if you think about it, you probably should do it. It's easier to revise a scar on the neck than to bring the dead back to life.

If you need an immediate surgical airway, then a **cricothyrotomy** is the preferred procedure if you aren't an experienced surgeon. It is easier and less bloody. Please remember the airway is best found in the neck by **palpation**, not inspection. Take a moment and palpate your own **cricothyroid membrane**, immediately below your **thyroid cartilage**. To do an emergency **cricothyrotomy** you need only a knife. Feel the space, cut down and stick your finger in the hole, feel, and cut again, and again until you are in the airway. Don't worry about bleeding. Place an **endotracheal tube** in the hole (again, by feel). Be sure not to push it past the **carina**. By this time, you will be shaking like a leaf—it's OK to let someone else squeeze the bag. Pressure with a dressing will address most bleeding. Occasionally, you might need to use some sutures to stop the bleeding.

Cholena Atresia is a congenital disorder where the nasal cholena is accluded by soft tissue, bone, or a combination of both. When unilateral it presents with unilateral mucoperialis discharge. When bilateral, the neonate is unable to breath. Since newborns are obligate nasal breathers, establishing an airway is an acute otolarynologic emergency. This can be done in the operating room.

Difficult Intubations:

Anatomic characteristics of the upper airway in some patients can result in difficult **laryngeal exposure**. Patients with **macroglossia** or **congenital micrognathia**, such as **Pierre Robin syndrome**, are examples. More commonly encountered is the young, muscular, overweight man with a short neck. Anesthesiologists are trained to recognize and manage the airway in these patients, but everyone caring for them must be aware of the potential difficulty. The need for a surgical airway in these patients often represents a failure of recognition and planning.

Ludwig's Angina and Deep Neck Infections:

Ludwig's angina is an infection in the floor of the mouth that causes the tongue to be pushed up and back, eventually obstructing the patient's airway. Treatment requires **incision and drainage of the abscess**. The most common cause of this abscess is infection in the teeth. The mylohyoid line on the inner aspect of the body of the **mandible** descends **on a slant** such that the tips of the roots of the **2nd and 3rd molars** are behind and below this line.

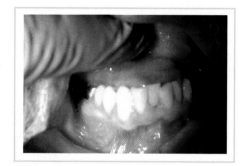

Figure 4.1.

This photograph depicts a gentleman with severe Ludwig's angina. Notice the swollen floor of the mouth and the arched protruding tongue obstructing the airway.

15

Therefore, if these teeth are abscessed, the pus will go into the **submandibular space** and may spread to the **parapharyngeal space**. These patients present with unilateral neck swelling, redness, pain, and fever. Usually, the infected tooth isn't painful. Treatment is incision and drainage over the submandibular swelling. Antibiotic coverage should include **oral cavity anaerobes**. If, however, the tooth roots are above the mylohyoid line, as they are from the **1st molar** forward, the infection will enter the **sublingual space**. This is above and in front of the mylohyoid and will cause the tongue to be pushed up and back, as previously noted. These patients usually will require tracheotomy, as the infection can progress quite rapidly, producing airway obstruction. The firm tongue swelling prevents standard laryngeal exposure with a **laryngoscope blade**, so **intubation** should not be attempted. Even if there is no airway obstruction on presentation, it may develop after you operate and drain the pus. This results because there is often **postoperative** swelling, which can be worse than the swelling on initial presentation.

Acute Supraglottic Swelling:

See chapter 17, Pediatric Otolaryngology.

This can occur as a result of infections (**epiglottitis**). It was once common in children, but is now rare because of the widespread utilization of vaccination against *Haemophilus influenzae*. Early recognition of the constellation of noisy breathing, high fever, drooling, and the characteristic posture, sitting upright with the jaw thrust forward, may be lifesaving. Epiglotic or supraglotic edema prevents swallowing. Relaxation and an upright position keeps the airway open. These children must not be examined until after the airway is secured.

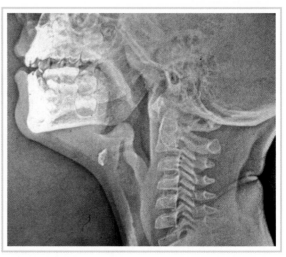

Figure 4.2.

Lateral neck, soft tissue x-ray of a child with acute epiglottitis. Note the lack of definition of the epiglottis, often referred to as a "thumb sign."

Angioneurotic edema, either familial or due to a **functional or quantitative deficiency of C1-esterase inhibitor**, can also result in dramatic swelling of the tongue, pharyngeal tissues, and the supraglottic airway. Swelling can progress rapidly, and oral intubation may quickly become impossible, urgently requiring a surgical airway.

16

Peritonsillar Abscess:

This is a collection of purulence in the space between the tonsil and the pharyngeal constrictor. Typically, the patient will have had an untreated sore throat for several days which has now gotten worse on one side. The hallmark signs of peritonsillar abscess are fullness of the anterior tonsillar pillar, uvular deviation away from the side of the abscess a "hot potato" voice and in some patients trismus (difficulty opening the jaws). Treatment includes drainage or aspiration, adequate pain control and antibiotics. Tonsillectomy may be indicated depending on the patients past history.

Foreign Bodies:

Foreign bodies can present as airway emergencies. Usually, however, by the time the patient gets to the emergency room, the foreign body in the airway has been expelled (often by the **Heimlich maneuver**) or else the patient is no longer able to be resuscitated. Foreign bodies in the **pharynx** or **laryngeal inlet** can often be extracted by **Magill forceps** after laryngeal exposure with a standard laryngoscope. The patient will usually vomit, so **suction is mandatory. Bronchial foreign bodies** will require operative **bronchoscopy** for removal. Occasionally a tracheotomy will be required, such as for a patient who has aspirated a partial denture with imbedded hooks.

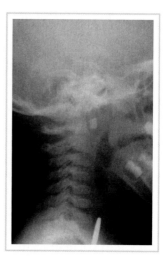

Figure 4.3.

A coin is seen here trapped in the patient's esophagus.

Children often aspirate peanuts, small toys, etc., into their bronchi. Occasionally these patients present as airway emergencies, although they more typically present with **unexplained cough or pneumonia**. Chevalier Jackson, the famous **bronchoscopist**, has noted, "All that wheezes is not asthma"—in other words, always remember to think of foreign body aspiration when a pediatric patient presents with unexplained cough or pneumonia. If a **ball-valve obstruction** results, **hyperinflation of the obstructed lobe or segment** can occur. This is easier to visualize on **inspiration-expiration films**.

17

Mucormycosis:

This is a **fungal infection** occurring in **immunocompromised** hosts. Typically it appears in patients receiving bone marrow transplantation or chemotherapy. It is a devastating disease, with a significant associated mortality. *Mucor* is a ubiquitous fungus that can become **invasive** in susceptible patients, classically diabetics with **poor glucose regulation** who became **acidotic**. If there is any other **system failure** (e.g., **renal failure**), mortality goes up significantly. The fungus grows in the blood vessels, causing **thrombosis** and **distal ischemia** and ultimately, tissue necrosis. This also leads to an **acid environment** in which the fungus thrives. The primary symptom is facial pain, and physical exam shows **black turbinates** due to **necrosis of the mucosa**. Diagnosis is made by **biopsy. Acutely branching nonseptate hyphae** are seen microscopically. Usually the infection starts in the sinuses but rapidly spreads to the **nose, eye, and palate**, and up the **optic nerve** to the **brain**.

Treatment is immediate correction of the **acidosis** and **metabolic stabilization** to the point where **general anesthesia** will be safely tolerated (usually for patients in **diabetic ketoacidosis [DKA]** who need several hours for rehydration, etc.). Then, wide **debridement**, usually consisting of a **medial maxillectomy** but often extending to a **radical maxillectomy** and **orbital exenteration** (removal of the eye and part of the hard palate) or even beyond. **Amphotericin B** is the drug of choice. Many patients have renal failure, which precludes adequate dosing. Newer **lysosomal forms** of amphotericin B have been shown to salvage these patients by permitting higher doses of drugs. If the underlying immunologic problem can't be arrested, survival is unlikely. In patients who are neutropenic, unless the white blood cell count improves, there is no chance for survival.

Acute Frontal or Sphenoid Sinusitis, and Cavernous Sinus Thrombosis:

See chapter 9, Rhinology, Nasal Obstruction and Sinusitis.

Epistaxis:

Epistaxis is common and occurs in all people at some time. If the condition is severe or persistent, these people become patients. The most common bleed is from the anterior part of the septum. This area has many blood vessels and is called **Kiesselbach's plexus**. In children, these nosebleeds should be treated with **oxymetazoline or phenylephrine** nose spray and digital **pressure for 5-10 minutes**. It is important for patients to look at the clock while applying the pressure: Just 30 seconds can seem like an hour in such a situation, and they may release the pressure too soon (which allows new blood to wash out the clot that was forming). The most common initiating event for these kinds of nosebleeds is **digital trauma** from a fingernail. Trim children's fingernails, and adults should be reminded to refrain. (These patients can even pick their nose during their sleep.) Another consideration may be an **occult bleeding disorder**; therefore, **adequate coagulation parameters** should be studied if the patient continues to have problems.

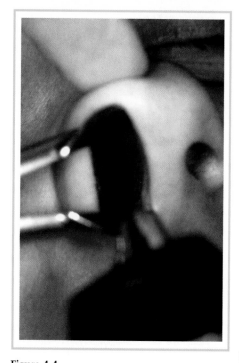

Figure 4.4.

Septal perforation may be secondary to trauma, cocaine (or even Afrin) abuse, or prior surgery. Epistaxis commonly accompanies this condition and may be problematic.

19

Recurrent nosebleeds in a teenager can be especially problematic. **Cocaine abuse** is always a possibility and must be considered. Very often in these cases, there will actually be a **perforation in the nasal septum**. Bleeding from the back of the nose in an adolescent male is considered to be a **juvenile nasopharyngeal angiofibroma** until proven otherwise. These patients also frequently have nasal obstruction. Diagnosis is made by physical examination with **nasal endoscopy**.

Some adult patients, often with HTN and **arthritis** (for which they are taking **aspirin**), have frequent nosebleeds. Whenever they present to the emergency room, they have a **significant elevation of blood pressure**, which isn't helped by the excitement of seeing a brisk nosebleed.

Treatment for these patients is **topical vasoconstriction** (oxymetazoline, phenylephrine). This almost always stops the bleeding. When the oxymetazoline-soaked pledgets are removed, a small red spot, which represents the source of the bleeding, can often be seen on the septum. Often, if such a bleeding source is seen, it can be **cauterized** with either **electric cautery** or **chemical cauterization with silver nitrate**. Nasal endoscopes permit identification of the bleeding site, even if it isn't immediately seen on the anterior septum. These patients should also be treated with medication to lower their blood pressure. The **diastolic pressure** has to be reduced **below 90 mm Hg**. Many patients can then go home, using oxymetazoline for a few days. Furthermore, methycellulose coated with antibiotic ointment can be placed into the nose to **prevent further trauma and allow the mucosal surfaces to heal**. This is usually left in place for 3-5 days. Sometimes the bleeding can't be completely stopped, and **packing** is then used as a **pressure method** of stopping the bleeding.

If the bleeding is coming from the **posterior aspect of the nose**, then a posterior pack may need to be placed. An alternative is to place any one of various commercially available balloons to stop the nosebleed. Patients who undergo anterior packing on one side may go home; however, if **bilateral nasal packing** is used or a posterior pack is placed, patients will need to be admitted to the hospital and carefully watched, because they can suffer from **hypoventilation** and **oxygen desaturation**. In general, the packing is left in place for 3-5 days and removed. During this time prophylactic oral or parenteral antibiotics should be administered to keep the smell down and decrease the infectious complications. If the patient rebleeds, the packing is replaced and **arterial ligation, endoscopic cautery, or embolization can be considered**.

As always, these patients should be worked up for **bleeding disorders**. A patient with a severe nosebleed can develop hypovolemia, or significant anemia, if fluid is being replaced. These conditions necessitate **increased cardiac output**, which can lead to ischemia or **infarction of the heart** itself.

Necrotizing Otitis Externa:

"**Malignant**" otitis externa is an old name for what should more appropriately be called **necrotizing otitis externa**. This is a **severe infection** of the external auditory canal, which is usually caused by *Pseudomonas* organisms. This infection spreads to the **temporal bone** and as such is really an **osteomyelitis** of the temporal bone. This can extend readily to the base of the skull, leading to fatal complications if it isn't adequately treated. This disease **occurs most commonly in diabetics,** and any patient with otitis externa should be asked about the possibility of diabetes. It can be caused by irrigating wax from the ears of diabetic patients. Usually these patients are elderly, and they present with **pain on the infected side and granulation tissue at the area of the bony cartilaginous junction in the external auditory canal.** To diagnose an actual infection in the bone (which is the sine qua non of this disease), a **computed tomography (CT)** scan of the bone, with bone windows, is obtained. A **technetium bone scan** will also demonstrate a "hot spot," but is too sensitive to discriminate between severe otitis externa and true osteomyelitis.

The standard therapy is **daily debridement of the external auditory canal, antipseudomonal ear drops**, and intravenous antipseudomonal antibiotics. **Quinolones** are the drugs of choice because they are active against *Pseudomonas* organisms.

Sudden Sensorineural Hearing Loss:

21

Sudden sensorineural hearing loss may occur for a variety of reasons, and most often the reason is unclear, but these patients recover their hearing much better if they are given high dose steroids (60 mg. of prednisone) tapered over about 3 weeks. The earlier the treatment starts, the better the prognosis, therefore **start the steroids immediately,** even if they can't be seen by an otolaryngologist for a day or so. Some evidence suggests that antivirals may also help slightly, so the patients are also given famcyclovir 500 mg. three times per day for 10 days. Recovery of some form can be expected in 2 out of 3 patients.

Questions, Section #4

1. Abscessed teeth can rupture through the medial mandibular cortex into the sublingual space. This can cause the tongue to be pushed up and back. The biggest danger in this is loss of _____.

2. The easiest way to ensure that the airway isn't lost in this situation is to perform a _____.

3. Immunocompromised patients, especially diabetics, can get a devastating fungal infection of the sinuses called _____.

4. When a frontal sinus air fluid level is seen on an x-ray, there is danger that the infection can readily spread through the veins that traverse the foramina of Brechet in the posterior wall and spread into the _____.

5. Necrotizing otitis externa is a *Pseudomonas* infection of the _____, which can lead to fatal complications.

6. Often, _____ tissue is seen at the junction of the bony-cartilaginous junction in the external auditory canal in patients with necrotizing otitis externa.

7. The most common cause of a nosebleed in children is injury to vessels in _____.

8. A posterior nosebleed in an adolescent male is considered to be a _____ until proven otherwise.

9. Two topical vasoconstrictors often used in the nose are _____ and _____.

10. In deciding between conflicting responsibilities, _____ should always be your first priority.

Answers

1. AIRWAY
2. TRACHEOTOMY
3. MUCORMYCOSIS
4. MENINGES
5. SKULL BASE OR TEMPORAL BONE
6. GRANULATION
7. KIESSELBACH'S PLEXUS
8. JUVENILE NASOPHARYNGEAL ANGIOFIBROMA
9. OXYMETAZOLINE, PHENYLEPHRINE
10. THE CARE OF THE PATIENT

The best preparation for tomorrow is to do today's work superbly well.

Sir William Osler

Otitis media may be thought of in terms of **Eustachian tube dysfunction**. You probably recognize the sensation of acute eustachian tube dysfunction due to a cold (upper respiratory infection [URI]) or allergy. If the tube

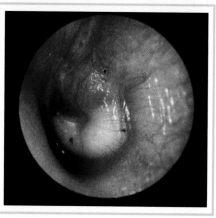

Figure 5.1.

This tympanic membrane demonstrates the bulging seen with an acute infection.

remains **obstructed**, **negative pressure** develops in the **middle ear** leading to **transudation of serous fluid**. When this is inoculated with **bacteria** from the **nasopharynx**, an acute otitis media develops. This is usually caused by *Streptococcus pneumoniae, Haemophilus influenzae*, or *Moraxella catarrhalis*. **First-line antibiotic therapy** is either amoxicillin or trimethoprim and sulfamethoxazole for 10 days. The high incidence of resistant organisms has made treatment of acute otitis media much more complicated. Failure to respond to first-line therapy is an indication for a second-line drug resistant to **beta-lactamase** and effective against resistant *Streptococcus* organisms. Treatment choices will be dictated by the prevalence of resistant organisms in your community. A **tympanocentesis** (ear tap) may be appropriate to obtain a culture, especially in immunocompromised patients, in regions where resistant *S. pneumoniae* are common, and in cases that fail to respond to standard therapy.

At 2 weeks, 50% of these patients will still have fluid in their ears. By 10 weeks, only about 10% will have residual fluid. In many children, the cycle then starts all over again, and they may have 5 or 6

23

bouts of acute otitis media in as many months. This is called **recurrent acute otitis media**.

These children benefit from **pressure equalization (PE) tube insertion**. Small tubes are placed in the **tympanic membrane (TM)** to "vent" the middle ear and prevent the negative pressure buildup in the first place. Note that the tube isn't intended to drain the fluid, but is for pressure equalization. If the ears drain after tubes have been inserted, the patient has otitis media. Children often grow out of the eustachian tube dysfunction by the time the tubes extrude on their own (1-2 years). Rarely a 3- to 6-month trial of antibiotic prophylaxis rec-

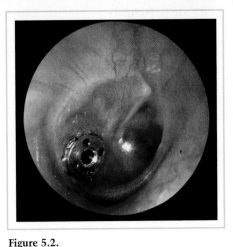

Figure 5.2.

Photograph of a tympanic membrane with a pressure equalizing (PE) tube in place. The tube permits aeration of the middle ear. It isn't intended for the drainage of fluid, as drainage through a PE tube represents infection.

ommended. This has been shown to **decrease the incidence** of recurrent acute otitis media, but **enhances the development of resistant organisms** and is controversial. If patients "break through" and have an episode while on prophylaxis, then tubes are indicated. You can **anticipate changes in practice recommendations over the next several years** due to the effect of prophylaxis on the development of resistant organisms.

A variant of acute otitis media occurs when blisters start to form on the outer surface of the tympanic membrane. This condition is **exquisitely painful** until the blisters burst. The condition is called **bullous myringitis** and these patients have such pain that they require very strong analgesics (hydrocone or oxycodone) as well as topical numbing ear drops containing benzocaine such as Auralgan. The pain usually arises quite quickly, and then subsides very quickly when the blisters burst. Antibiotic treatment is the same as for acute otitis media.

Children with chronic eustachian tube dysfunction also develop **fluid without active infection**. Their eustachian tubes don't ventilate the

Only the curious will learn and only the resolute will overcome the obstacles to learning. The quest quotient has always excited me more than the intelligence quotient.

Eugene S. Wilson

middle ear space, and the fluid remains there without infection. This is **otitis media with effusion (OME)**. These patients may have up to a **30 decibel (dB) conductive hearing loss**. The hearing loss **affects speech development and learning**. Patients are often treated with antibiotics (even though the fluid isn't actually infected) because some studies show that such treatment will **clear up to 50% of the cases**. The idea is to **decrease the swelling** in the eustachian tube and **allow ventilation**. If the child is old enough, try to get him or her to "clear" the ears (**politzerization**) several times per day. If all these measures fail and hearing loss persists, then PE tubes should be placed. Treatment guidelines have been formalized that recommend placement of PE tubes if hearing loss persists for more than 3 months. An **adenoidectomy** is performed at the same time if the patient is getting his or her 2nd set of tubes. This usually prevents the re-accumulation of fluid in the ears. Children usually grow out of the need for the tubes as the eustachian tube assumes its longer and more downward slanted course with time.

OME in an adult, especially if it is **of recent duration and unilateral**, suggests a **disease process in the nasopharynx. Early nasopharyngeal carcinoma** is well known for its silent nature—usually the only sign is unilateral OME. Later in the disease process, the tumor **metastasizes to** the cervical lymph nodes and extends into the skull base, causing **cranial neuropathies**.

Nasopharyngeal examination is **mandatory** for any adult patient with unilateral OME. In the past, this was performed with mirrors, but most otolaryngologists now routinely use rigid and flexible endoscopic instrumentation.

Complications of Acute Otitis Media:

Complications of acute otitis media were common in the pre-antibiotic era. It is largely because of those complications that otolaryngology developed as a specialty more than 100 years ago. Most physicians practicing today have never seen a case of **mastoiditis** or **meningitis** due to otitis media. However, **as the prevalence of resistant organisms increases**, especially *Streptococcal pneumoniae*, there is a chance that **these complications may become more common**. Therefore, even if you never see a case during your medical school years, you must know about these complications and be able to recognize them should you encounter them in your practice.

If untreated, acute otitis media can lead to **several complications**, one of which is **perforation of the eardrum**. **Purulence** must drain someplace, and this is the path of least resistance in the ear. Treatment is with both systemic and topical antibiotics, quinolones are the optimal choice; currently **ofloxacin otic solution (0.3%)** is the only topical agent approved for use in the presence of a tympanic membrane perforation. The perforation will often heal on its own; however, if it doesn't, this can lead to chronic otitis media, which by definition refers to a hole in the TM. Also, a **particularly severe infection can necrose the long process of the incus** by cutting off the blood supply. Although this occurs more commonly with a **cholesteatoma**, it can also occur with an acute infection. Another **residual effect** of acute otitis media can be **tympanosclerosis**, firm submucosal scarring that can appear as a chalky white patch on the TM. It can **infrequently lead to conductive hearing loss if the middle ear and ossicles are involved**

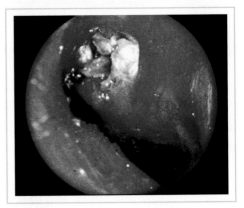

Figure 5.3.

Otoscopic view of left eardrum with cholesteatoma involving the pars flaccida. The white material is keratin filling the canal.

extensively. Other complications of acute otitis media are more severe. Meningitis, for example, is felt to occur by **blood-borne spread** of the bacteria into the **meninges**. The most common offending organism for this was *Haemophilus influenzae*, though epidemiologic patterns may change with the advent of the *Haemophilus influenzae* vaccine. Of academic interest is that the method of spread to the meninges in **frontal sinusitis** is felt to be direct extension of **thrombophlebitis**, but in otologic complications, it is felt to be blood borne.

Infection of the air cells in the mastoid just behind the ear occurs when acute otitis media is present. However, if **the infection becomes more severe and invades the bony structures**, it becomes acute mastoiditis. The condition presents as **ear pain** associated with a **draining**

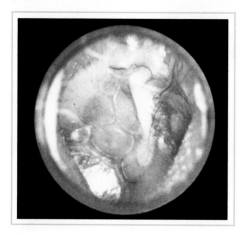

Figure 5.4.

Photograph of a tympanic membrane with chronic otitis media with effusion (COME). Note the bubbles in the fluid behind the drum. This is a common condition that affects children. Most will respond spontaneously and will not require surgical intervention.

perforated eardrum. Remember that once the TM has **ruptured**, in acute otitis media there is **no pain**. If pain develops, usually 1 or 2 weeks later, you must consider mastoiditis. A CT scan is a useful diagnostic tool. The condition may resolve with intravenous antibiotics; however, it **may also require surgical drainage of the mastoid**. The complications of mastoiditis are legendary. Sometimes, a collection of pus can occur just outside the **dura**, termed an **epidural abscess**, and surgical drainage is required. The **sigmoid sinus can become infected, thrombose**, and serve as a **nidus of infection**. This classically leads to **showers of infected emboli**, causing "**picket fence fevers**." **Brain abscesses** can also occur as a result of acute otitis media, as can facial nerve paralysis. The **facial nerve paralysis** is felt to be due to **inflammation** around the nerve, and this generally responds to appropriate intravenous antibiotic therapy as well as drainage of the pus, through either a **myringotomy** or, if necessary, a **mastoidectomy**. It is possible that these complications, now rare, may become more common in the future.

Some people don't outgrow their eustachian tube dysfunction. They may suffer from chronic negative middle ear pressure. This can **retract part of the pars flaccida** of the TM back into the middle ear. The outside of the TM is lined with **squamous epithelium**, which **desquamates**. Over the course of time, the **keratinous debris** can get caught in the pars flaccida pocket. This can continue to accumulate, expanding the pocket, and is then called a cholesteatoma, which often gets infected. The patients may be put on **antibiotic/steroid drops** and their drainage may get better, only to come back when the treatment is stopped. If the cholesteatoma is left untreated, it will **continue to grow and erode bony structures.** Possible sequelae include **hearing loss secondary to necrosis**

of the long process of the incus due to pressure on a bone with a tenuous blood supply, **erosion into the lateral semicircular canal** causing dizziness, **subperiosteal abscess, facial nerve palsy**, meningitis, and brain abscess.

The treatment of cholesteatoma is surgical removal. They aren't cancers and don't metastasize. Remember that excision gets rid of the cholesteatoma, but not the eustachian tube dysfunction and sometimes these recur. A PE tube will prevent chronic negative middle ear pressure. Once patients have undergone surgery for removal of a cholesteatoma, they will need continuous monitoring of their ear for the rest of their life.

A cholesteatoma also can occur when squamous epithelium migrates into the middle ear space through a hole in the TM. The hole can come from a previous severe necrotizing infection, a previous PE tube hole that didn't heal, or trauma. **Marginal perforations are more likely to allow migration than central ones.** Remember that the TM has **3 layers: cuboidal epithelium in the middle ear, a fibrous layer, and squamous epithelium on the outside.** When there is a perforation, all 3 layers start to **proliferate**, but if the **squamous layer and the cuboidal layer meet**, the **fibrous layer will stop**. This can lead to a chronic perforation.

By definition, "chronic otitis media" means "TM perforation." The logic behind this older nomenclature is that the middle ear is constantly being exposed to the outside and has a low-grade inflammation chronically associated with it. Curiously, a **perforation usually doesn't cause much of a hearing loss.** In fact, even if the entire TM is gone, the hearing loss is only about 40 dB.

Clinical Example:

A 14-year-old comes to your office complaining of painless right ear drainage. He is otherwise healthy, although he did have PE tubes in his ears as a child. On examination, you find he has slightly turbid drainage coming from a hole in his right TM. You diagnose chronic otitis media and learn that he doesn't know he has a perforation. He hasn't been trying to keep water out of his ear. You assume he has a *Pseudomonas aeruginosa* infection and prescribe **ofloxacin otic solution (0.3%)** b.i.d. for 10 days. He returns in 2 weeks with a dry ear and a small residual TM perforation. What test do you order next? An **audiogram**, which shows a 15 dB **conductive hearing loss with normal discrimination** (ability to understand words). You tell the patient to keep water out of his ear. He comes back in 4-6 weeks and hasn't had any more drainage, so you refer him for a **tympanoplasty (repair of the hole in the TM)**.

Tympanoplasty:

Tympanoplasty, an operation to patch a hole in the eardrum, is done in a way you might not expect. It is generally performed **through the ear canal or from behind the ear**. The surgeon freshens up the edges of the hole (where the squamous layer has crossed over the fibrous layer and met the cuboidal layer). Then, because the fibrous tissue won't grow with squamous epithelium meeting cuboidal epithelium, a piece of **fascia temporalis** or **tragal perichondrium** is harvested as a **graft**. Small, semicircular cuts in the skin of the **external auditory canal (EAC)** are made about 5 mm out from the **annulus**. The surgeon scrapes the skin off the bone and sneaks under the annulus to the **medial aspect** of the TM. The middle ear is then filled with a sponge-like material made of hydrolyzed collagen, which acts as a scaffold holding the graft up against the medial aspect of the eardrum. Then the TM and skin are replaced and the EAC is packed. The collagen substance is eventually reabsorbed; meanwhile, the fibrous layer proliferates along the scaffolding of the graft to close the hole. We usually leave the ear alone for 3 weeks, then gently suction out any remaining collagen substance from the EAC.

Let's say a 49-year-old, male, nondiabetic comes to your clinic with a draining right ear. He says it has drained off and on for years. Once again, the ENT exam is normal except for copious purulence coming out of a TM perforation. You give him ciprofloxacin, 500 mg, orally BID and **ofloxacin otic solution (0.3%)** ear drops BID. You tell him to keep water out of his ear, which he does, and he comes back in 2 weeks, cleared up. You order an audiogram, which shows a 20 dB conductive hearing loss and good discrimination. He is then scheduled for a tympanoplasty in 6 weeks, but he comes in draining again in 2 weeks. He hasn't gotten his ear wet. You repeat medical therapy and, once again, he clears but drains a month later. He has a deep nidus of infection in his mastoid cavity that needs to be cleared. You schedule him for a CT scan, which shows no cholesteatoma, and then you perform a **tympanomastoidectomy**. At surgery, you find normal air cells throughout the mastoid cavity, with the exception of a few infected cells at the very tip of the mastoid. He does well postop.

Now, let's say you have the same history and you couldn't see a cholesteatoma by physical exam (you almost never can), but the CT scan shows it. The audio is the same. You perform the same operation (a tympanomastoidectomy) and remove the cholesteatoma. The patient does well postop. Did you notice that when patients present with a recurrent draining ear, appropriate therapy includes systemic antibiotics as well as antibiotic-containing topical eardrops? This includes patients who have a previously placed PE tube. Currently, there is a trend to use quinilone drops such as **ofloxacin otic solution (0.3%)** rather than neomycin-containing preparations due to the theoretical risk of neomycin-induced inner ear damage.

Drops alone are needed for uncomplicated **otitis externa (swimmer's ear)**. *P. aeruginosa* is the bug here, and it doesn't do well in an acidic environment. That is why many swimmers use half-strength vinegar for prevention. Remember: The sine qua non of otitis externa is **pain on traction of the pinna**. Tragal compression may also elicit discomfort. If you pull on the ear and it doesn't increase the pain, the patient doesn't have otitis externa. If the EAC swells shut, you insert a small sponge, which wicks the drops down into the ear canal. Remember also that in diabetic patients, the infection can progress to necrotizing otitis externa.

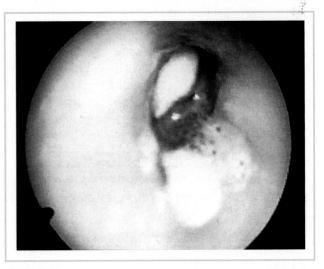

Figure 5.5.

Fungal otitis externa. The white areas that resemble cotton are fungal filaments.

Questions, Section #5

1. The most common organisms causing otitis media are
    _____, _____, and _____.

2. The length of time acute otitis media should be treated for is
    _____.

3. _____ % of children with acute otitis media that have
    been adequately treated will still have fluid in their ears at 2 weeks.

4. _____ % of children with successfully treated acute
    otitis media will have residual fluid in their ears at 10 weeks.

5. The presence of bilateral fluid in the ears may cause up to a
    _____dB conductive hearing loss.

6. It is important to examine the _____ in
    any adult with unilateral otitis media with effusion.

7. PE tubes are not placed to drain fluid from the middle ear. They
    serve to_____the ear.

8. The first thing you look at on an x-ray is_____.

9. The secret to becoming a good physician is to _____ for
    1 hour every day.

10. The collection of trabeculated bony cavities lined with mucosa and
    connected with the middle ear are called the mastoid
    _____.

11. The pars flaccida of the TM can become _____ when
    there is chronic negative pressure in the middle ear.

12. The outside of the TM, including the pars flaccida, is lined with
    _____epithelium.

13. In the natural course of things, squamous epithelium tends to lose
    the stratum _____.

14. As the stratum corneum desquamates off of a retracted pars flacci-
    da, sometimes it can't easily reach the external auditory canal. If
    this occurs, the desquamated debris consisting mainly of keratin
    collects in the retracted pars flaccida. Over time, this can grow and
    become a _____.

15. When surgically removing a cholesteatoma, it is important to remove all _____epithelium that may have been retracted into the middle ear.

16. Desquamated epithelium can be a nidus of _____ in the middle ear.

17. If a patient presents with a draining ear, appropriate therapy includes drops and _____.

Answers

1. S. PNEUMONIAE, H. INFLUENZAE, M. CATARRHALIS
2. 10 DAYS
3. 50
4. 10
5. 30
6. NASOPHARYNX
7. VENT
8. THE NAME
9. READ
10. AIR CELLS
11. RETRACTED
12. SQUAMOUS
13. CORNEUM
14. CHOLESTEATOMA
15. SQUAMOUS
16. INFECTION
17. ANTIBIOTICS

People suffer from hearing loss for a wide variety of reasons. Patients may present with the complaint of being unable to hear, or they may complain of difficulty understanding. Often, a family member brings the patient for a hearing test because of difficulties in communication. Older individuals often complain of **tinnitus**, which may be described as a sound like "ringing," "buzzing," or "crickets" in the ears. Tinnitus is usually a manifestation of hearing loss, although it may have other causes as well. Hearing loss in children may be particularly difficult to detect, and is often confused with inattention or speech delay.

It is important to determine whether the problem is with the **conductive pathway of the ear** or with the **inner ear** or **8th cranial nerve**. **Conductive hearing loss** can be due to **cerumen impaction**, swelling of the external auditory canal, tympanic membrane perforations, middle ear fluid, or **ossicular chain abnormalities. Sensorineural hearing loss** can occur as a result of injury to the hair cells in the **cochlea** or neural elements innervating the hair cells. The most common etiologic factors are persistent noise exposure, age-related changes of the 8th cranial nerve **(presbycusis)**, familial or genetic factors, infectious or postinflammatory processes. Tumor growth along the course of the 8th cranial nerve can also be the etiology of sensorineural loss and must be included in the differential diagnosis. Treatment of these different types of hearing loss can be dramatically different.

Pure tone audiometry ("the hearing test") is frequently used to assess the patient's hearing levels. The test requires that the patient is able to, and wishes to cooperate (difficult in very young children). Hearing threshold levels are determined between 250 and 8000 **hertz (Hz)** for pure tones and measured in decibels (dB). The 0 dB level is "normalized" to young, healthy adults and doesn't mean there is absence of detectable sound. Some patients hear 0 decibels. To reach the threshold of hearing usually requires louder test signals. The higher the threshold is, the poorer the patient's hearing. Thresholds higher than 25 dB are considered abnormal.

During the **audiogram**, independent thresholds are determined for each ear for both **air conduction (conductive hearing)** and **bone conduction (sensorineural hearing)**. Air conduction measures the ability of the external and middle ear to transmit sound to the cochlea. Any blockage to sound transmission in this pathway (cerumen, perforation, middle ear fluid) will create an **air-bone gap**

between the air and bone conduction thresholds on the audiogram, and is an example of a conductive hearing loss.

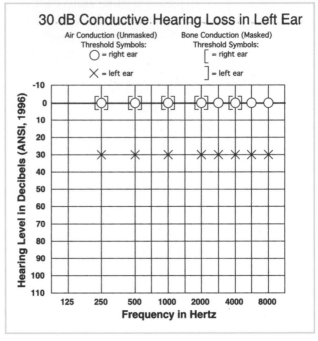

Figure 6.1.

A conductive hearing loss in the left ear due to otitis media with effusion. Note that bone conduction thresholds on both ears are normal but that air conduction on the left is 30 dB poorer than that measured on the right. Zero (0) dB doesn't refer to absence of sound, but rather represents an average of thresholds for young, healthy adults.

However, if the air conduction and bone conduction thresholds are equal but higher than 25 dB, this is called a sensorineural hearing loss.

Our ability to hear is more complex than just listening to single pure tones in a sound-proof booth. Therefore, a test of the patient's ability to understand spoken words is done as well. This is tested by presenting phonetically balanced words (love, boat, pool, sell, raise) into the audiogram, reported as the **speech discrimination** score (90-100% is normal). This test of clarity also assesses the function of the auditory division of the 8th cranial nerve. The ability to understand speech is very important, especially with respect to determining to what degree a hearing aid will help a particular patient. **Amplifying** garbled speech (with a hearing aid) has limited benefit for patients with very poor speech discrimination.

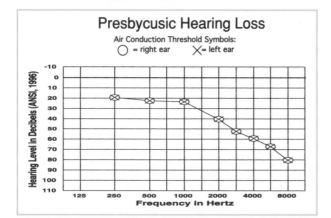

Figure 6.2.

Audiogram of a patient with presbycusis. Note that low tone thresholds are relatively normal with a drop in thresholds at higher frequencies. This is a consequence of the normal aging process and may vary widely from patient to patient.

Tympanometry is commonly used to evaluate the tympanic membrane and middle ear status. This test assesses the mobility of the tympanic membrane and its response to pressure changes in the external auditory canal. Three common patterns are shown in figure 6.4. **Type A** plots are present when the external auditory canal is patent and the middle ear and tympanic membrane are healthy (maximum TM mobility when pressure in the canal is atmospheric). **Type B** plots occur when the middle ear is filled with fluid or the tympanic membrane has a perforation (no peak in eardrum mobility). **Type C** plots (peak eardrum mobility when pressure is subatmospheric) are very typical of patients with retracted tympanic membranes secondary to eustachian tube dysfunction. Tympanometry can help in the detection of middle ear fluid when the physical exam is unclear.

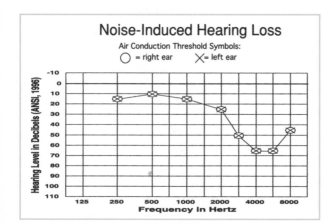

Figure 6.3.

Audiogram of a patient who has been exposed to noise. Note the high frequency dip, with a maximum loss at 4000 hertz. This audiogram suggests noise exposure that may be encountered occasionally in younger individuals who have been exposed to hazardous or "toxic" noise.

Conductive Hearing Loss:

Careful physical examination of the ear with the aid of a microscope, tuning fork tests, and audiometric testing can frequently determine the cause of a conductive hearing loss. Swelling of the external auditory canal secondary to otitis externa can be treated with appropriate topical medication. Cerumen impaction can be cleaned with specialized instru-

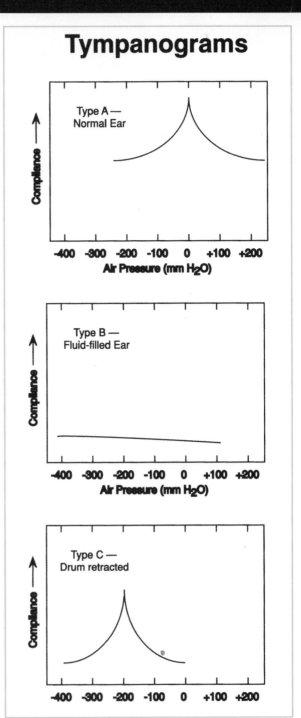

Tympanograms

Type A — Normal Ear

Type B — Fluid-filled Ear

Type C — Drum retracted

36

Figure 6.4.

Three tympanograms demonstrating change in compliance of the middle ear (vertical axis) with changes in ear canal pressure. Type A is normal, with the greatest compliance at the point where the pressure in the ear canal is equal to that of atmospheric pressure (peak is at 0). Type B demonstrates very poor compliance at any frequency, suggestive of a tympanic membrane immobilized by fluid in the middle ear (no peak). Type C represents a tympanogram in which the compliance of the membrane is greatest at a point where the pressure in the canal is 200 mm of water below that of atmospheric pressure (peak shifted to the left). This suggests inefficient eustachian tube function with persistent negative pressure in the middle ear.

ments. Middle ear fluid is a common cause of hearing loss in children and can be treated with antibiotic therapy or myringotomy tubes, and tympanic membrane perforations can be surgically repaired. Cholesteatoma often presents with hearing loss, and in the physical examination, it can be confused with cerumen. Conductive hearing loss present on the audiogram and is not readily apparent on the physical exam suggests problems with the ossicular chain. One common disease process affecting the ossicular chain is **otosclerosis**. This is a hereditary disease process that involves **bony proliferation within the temporal bone**. These bony changes commonly occur at the footplate region of the **stapes**, causing gradual fixation of the ossicular chain. This fixation **decreases the mobility** of the stapes footplate and creates a conductive hearing loss. Surgical correction—**stapedectomy**—is available. This procedure involves removing the fixed stapes ossicle and placing a prosthesis between the **incus** and the **vestibule of the inner ear**, which re-establishes **ossicular continuity**. Sound vibrations can then be transmitted from the ossicular chain into the inner ear through the prosthesis and restore the patient's hearing.

Sensorineural Hearing Loss:

Sensorineural hearing loss is the most common form of hearing loss. Causes of this type of hearing loss are quite varied. However, age-related changes to the cochlea causing presbycusis are by far the most frequent cause. As we age, the outer hair cells within the cochlea gradually deteriorate, causing a **symmetrical** sensorineural hearing loss that begins in the high frequencies (figure 6.2). Patients with presbycusis may also have difficulty with speech discrimination ability and complain of tinnitus. Another common type of hearing loss is secondary to **acoustic trauma** or "noise exposure." Noise exposure is common in certain industries and is closely regulated by a federal government agency, the Occupational Health and Safety Administration (OSHA). Recreational target shooting, hunting with firearms, use of personal stereos with headphones, loud music exposure, power tools, etc., can cause a specific type of hearing loss with a characteristic audiometric pattern (figure 6.3). Patients suffering from noise-induced hearing loss have a symmetric "noise notch" in bone conduction thresholds at approximately 4000 Hz. Treatment consists of hearing education, noise avoidance if possible, and appropriate hearing protection with ear plugs or ear muffs when loud noise is present. Prevention is

37

vital, and counseling should be part of routine health maintenance. Patients should also have regularly scheduled audiometric follow up.

Patients with **asymmetric** sensorineural hearing loss require a more thorough evaluation to rule out a benign tumor of the 8th cranial nerve known as an **acoustic neuroma**. Although most patients with an asymmetric hearing loss do not have an acoustic neuroma, hearing loss is by far the most common presenting complaint in patients with such tumors. In addition, these patients will frequently have very poor speech discrimination scores and tinnitus in the affected ear. They may also occasionally have disequilibrium complaints, although true **vertigo** is rare. Specialized audiometric testing can be done to assist in the diagnosis of acoustic neuromas, but magnetic resonance imaging (MRI) with gadolinium is now the gold-standard diagnostic test of choice.

Physical exam and testing may elucidate an easily treatable cause of hearing loss. However, more serious causes can be present that require careful assessment and complex management. Patients with hearing loss should be referred to an otolaryngologist for evaluation and management of their care. Many states require an evaluation by a physician before a hearing aid can be fitted, to ensure that diagnoses of such serious conditions as cholesteatoma or acoustic neuromas aren't missed.

Hearing aids are effective in rehabilitation of hearing loss in most patients. Aids vary widely in their power (gain), frequency response, size, and cost. Optimal fitting requires a professional knowledgeable in the nuances of amplification technology. For some patients with total sensorineural hearing loss, a cochlear implant provides direct stimulation of the cochlear nerve and is very helpful. Currently patients with bilateral profound hearing loss are candidates. We are able to implant younger and younger children as well, which has proven extremely helpful in their language and social development. All newborns should undergo hearing screening, so appropriate measures may be taken as soon as possible.

Questions, Section #6

1. The most common cause of a conductive hearing loss in children is _____.

2. The most common cause of conductive hearing loss in adults is
    _____.

3. The magnitude of a hearing loss is documented in the
    _____.

4. The two major types of hearing loss are _____ and
    _____.

5. Conductive hearing loss is present when there is a difference between _____and _____conduction thresholds.

6. Sensorineural hearing loss is present when abnormal air and bone conduction thresholds _____ one another.

7. Noise-induced hearing loss often produces a high-frequency _____ in the audiogram.

8. Otitis media with effusion produces a _____ tympanogram.

9. Presbycusis produces a hearing loss that slopes _____ to the _____ side of the audiogram.

10. A patient with an asymmetric sensorineural hearing loss must be evaluated for the potential of having an _____.

11. Any facial paralysis of gradual onset, delayed (greater than 2 months) recovery, or that recurs requires further evaluation of the facial nerve with a _____.

Answers
1. FLUID IN THE MIDDLE EAR (OTITIS MEDIA W/EFFUSION)
2. CERUMEN IMPACTION
3. AUDIOGRAM
4. CONDUCTIVE, SENSORINEURAL
5. AIR, BONE
6. APPROXIMATE
7. NOTCH
8. TYPE B (FLAT)
9. DOWNWARD, RIGHT
10. ACOUSTIC NEUROMA
11. GADOLINIUM-ENHANCED MRI SCAN

Dizziness

People often come to the ENT doctor with a complaint of dizziness. Many symptoms, such as dysequilibrium, **syncope**, lightheadedness, **ataxia**, and vertigo, are commonly described as "dizziness." As otolaryngologists, we focus on disease processes that produce true vertigo (an illusion of motion), which is primarily associated with the balance organs of the inner ear. If your patient doesn't complain of true illusion of motion, redirect your questioning to evaluation of syncope or **episodic hypotension**.

Vestibular Neuronitis:

One of the most common causes of vertigo is **vestibular neuronitis**. It is thought to be caused by inflammation of the **vestibular portion of the 8th cranial nerve** or of the inner ear balance organs (**vestibular labyrinth**). Another term for this entity is **labyrinthitis**. It is thought that the condition is secondary to a viral infection, and it is frequently associated with recent flu symptoms (upper respiratory infection). The patient will usually awaken with room-spinning vertigo that will gradually become less intense over 24-48 hours. During this period, the patient's hearing is generally unchanged, and it may take weeks for the symptoms to completely resolve. Nausea with or without emesis is not unusual. Treatment is symptomatic including **vestibular suppressant medication**, antiemetic medication, and a short, tapering course of oral steroids. **Residual vestibulopathy** that persists for months or years isn't uncommon, and is best managed with vestibular exercises.

Benign Paroxysmal Positional Vertigo (BPPV):

Another common cause of vertigo seen by otolaryngologists is **BPPV**. This disorder is caused by **otoconia (calcium carbonate crystals)** or other sediment that have become free floating and enter one of the balance canals. When the patient turns his or her head quickly or into a certain position, this free-floating material moves the balance canal

Figure 7.1.

Bedside maneuver for the treatment of a patient with benign paroxysmal positional vertigo (BPPV) affecting the right ear. The presumed position of the debris within the labyrinth during the maneuver is shown in panels A-D. The maneuver is a 3-step procedure. The Dix-Hallpike test is performed with the patient's head rotated 45° toward the right ear, and the neck slightly extended with the chin pointed slightly upward. This position results in the patient's head hanging to the right (panel A). Once the vertigo and the nystagmus provoked by the Dix-Hallpike test cease, the patient's head is rotated about the rostral-caudal body axis until the left ear is down (panel B). Then the head and body are further rotated until the head is face down (panel C). The vertex of the head is kept tilted downward throughout the rotation. The maneuver usually provokes brief vertigo. The patient should be kept in the final, facedown position for about 10-15 seconds. With the head kept turned toward the left shoulder, the patient is brought into the seated position (panel D). Once the patient is upright, the head is tilted so that the chin is pointed slightly downward.

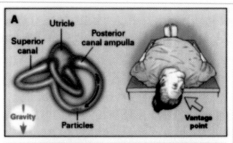

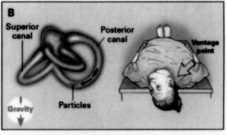

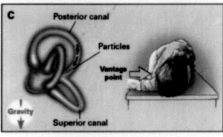

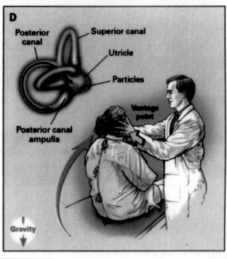

fluid (**endolymph**) and stimulates the vestibular division of the 8th cranial nerve. This motion creates an intense feeling of vertigo that lasts less than 30 seconds and passes when the material settles in place. Patients are usually able to describe the precise motion that precipitates this intense, brief episode of vertigo. Rolling over in bed is a move-

41

ment that frequently initiates an episode. The name of the syndrome is related to the intense, episodic (paroxysmal) vertigo initiated by certain head positions (positional) that isn't related to a **central nervous system (CNS)** tumor (benign).

This disorder can occur without any specific inciting event, but is often seen after significant head trauma or an episode of vestibular neuronitis. BPPV can be successfully treated with a particle repositional maneuver in the office setting. Dislodged, free-floating sediment that has entered the balance organs can be repositioned into the vestibule (portion of the inner ear) by rolling the patient 270 degrees from the supine position. Medical therapy with vestibular suppressants is ineffective (because the episodes of vertigo are so fleeting) and should be discouraged.

Ménière's Disease:

Ménière's disease is classically diagnosed by history because patients have a particular symptom complex. Patients develop intense, episodic vertigo, usually lasting from 30 minutes to 2-4 hours and associated with fluctuating hearing loss, roaring tinnitus, and the sensation of aural fullness. (Remember that in BPPV, the vertigo lasts less than 1 minute, and in vestibular neuronitis, the vertigo lasts 24-48 hours.) Although the precise cause of Ménière's disease hasn't been unequivocally determined, the symptoms are believed to be secondary to a distention of the **endolymphatic** space within the balance organs of the inner ear. The disease can be very difficult to treat because its course is very unpredictable. Patients can suffer from frequent attacks and then abruptly stop having symptoms, only to resume attacks years later. Treatment strategies have been focused on decreasing the endolymphatic fluid pressure within the vestibular portion of the inner ear. Salt restriction and thiazide diuretics are frequently used as first-line agents. If this doesn't adequately control the patient's symptoms, additional intervention can be used. **Vestibular ablation by instillation of ototoxic medication** (i.e., gentamicin) into the middle ear for inner ear absorption through the round window membrane has also been used with success, and has a low incidence of hearing loss. Surgical options for incapacitated patients include **endolymphatic sac decompression into the mastoid cavity**, vestibular nerve section, and **labyrinthectomy.** Vestibular nerve section involves transecting the vestibular portion of the 8th cranial nerve near the brainstem and requires an intracranial procedure. This procedure disrupts the aberrant vestibular signals from the affected ear while preserving the patient's current hearing thresholds. If the patient has had Ménière's disease for an extended length of time, the hearing has usually declined to the point of not being useful. Labyrinthectomy is then considered because this procedure also disrupts the aberrant vestibular signals but destroys any hearing in the operated ear. It avoids the risks associated with an intracranial surgical procedure. Treatment of patients with Ménière's disease must be managed in a step-wise fashion with careful consideration given to the patient's intensity of symptoms and frequency of attacks, as well as how the disease is affecting his or her life and overall general health. Medical and surgical treatments are effective and are preferable to disability.

Questions, Section #7

1. Dizziness associated with an illusion of motion is termed
   _____.

2. Sudden vertigo that develops without ear symptoms and lasts for
   24-48 hours is most likely_____.

3. BPPV or_____is vertigo
   characteristically precipitated by positional changes, lasts 10-30
   seconds, and isn't associated with serious illness.

Answers

1. VERTIGO
2. VESTIBULAR NEURONITIS OR LABYRINTHITIS
3. BENIGN PAROXYSMAL POSITIONAL VERTIGO

Facial paralysis is a devastating condition for the patient and his or her family. It may occur spontaneously, following trauma or surgical procedure, or as a result of malignant tumors of the pinna, the parotid gland, or the skull base. Paralysis involving all divisions of the nerve is **peripheral**, and that sparing the forehead is **central**. Facial paralysis is usually graded on a scale of 1 to 6, where 1 is normal and 6 is a flaccid complete paralysis.

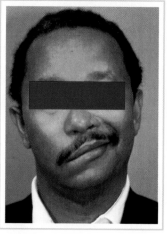

Figure 8.1.

This patient has suffered paralysis of the right facial nerve, hence the asymmetry when he attempts to smile. Facial nerve paralysis involves both the upper and lower divisions of the facial nerve. A lesion of the supranuclear tracts would spare the forehead and represent a "central 7th."

45

Bell's Palsy:

Bell's palsy is a unilateral facial nerve paralysis that is, by definition, **idiopathic**. You must be careful to rule out other potential causes of facial paralysis before making this diagnosis.

Polymerase chain reaction (PCR) studies have demonstrated herpetic infection in a majority of cases. Therefore, a better term might be **viral or herpetic facial paralysis**.

The clinical course of Bell's palsy is quite characteristic. The onset is usually sudden, with the patient often noticing the symptoms upon waking from sleep. The recovery is gradual, but spontaneous recovery can be expected in more than 85% of the cases. Medical therapy (within 3 days) with oral steroids (60 mg of prednisone) and antiviral medication acyclovir or famciclovir has been shown to decrease the incidence of incomplete recovery. Careful history taking is important in treating these patients. **Gradual onset** of symptoms (over months), paralysis that doesn't begin to recover by several months, or **recurrent** symptoms on the same side suggest tumor and should be further **evaluated** by gadolinium-enhanced MRI. Studies have shown that up to 30% of patients diagnosed with idiopathic Bell's palsy were found to have another cause for their facial paralysis, such as a facial nerve neuroma, parotid gland malignancy, or **cerebello-pontine angle tumor**.

Ramsay-Hunt's Syndrome:

Another syndrome that includes facial nerve paralysis is Ramsay-Hunt's or **herpes zoster oticus**. Facial nerve paralysis is accompanied by severe pain and a vesicular eruption in the external auditory canal and auricle in the distribution of the facial nerve. The vesicular lesions generally precede the facial nerve paralysis, but this isn't always the case. Vesicles may be nonpainful, quite small, or even undetectable. The prognosis for recovery is significantly poorer than in Bell's palsy. Medical therapy with antiviral agents and oral steroids is now considered standard and should be instituted early in the course of the disorder.

Temporal Bone Fractures:

The facial nerve has an elongated course throughout the temporal bone. Significant head trauma producing fracture lines through the temporal bone can affect the facial nerve in one of two ways. The fracture line can directly traverse the facial nerve and transect it or cause a bony fragment to directly impale the nerve, or the fracture line may be some distance away from the nerve but cause stretching or bruising of the nerve. This second situation creates edema and swelling of the nerve and its surrounding sheath, which can impede axoplasmic flow and create a conduction block. Unless the facial nerve has been completely transected, the swelling and subsequent facial nerve paralysis can take up to 72 hours to develop. Therefore, careful assessment of the facial nerve **at initial presentation** is important in later management decisions. Unfortunately, the patient has usually suffered significant head trauma and may have multiple other injuries that render him or her unconscious and unable to perform voluntary facial motion. Also, medical teams may be performing lifesaving intervention, with facial nerve assessment not an immediate priority. If the status of the facial nerve is in question, specialized electrical testing and high-resolution CT scanning of the temporal bone can be done to assess the facial nerve along its intratemporal course. If the nerve appears to be impaled by a bony spicule, facial nerve exploration via a transmastoid and/or intracranial approach should be done. Facial nerve transection can be repaired with either direct **reanastomosis** or with an **interposition graft (greater auricular or sural nerve)** if undue tension would occur with reanastomosis. Most facial nerve injuries related to trauma involve contusion injuries that can be followed expectantly and tend to do well over the long term.

Temporal bone trauma can also affect a patient's hearing. If the fracture line disrupts the cochlea or balance organs, a complete sensorineural hearing loss is frequently seen. However, if the fracture involves the middle ear or ear canal, conductive hearing loss may occur secondary to a middle ear blood collection (**hemotympanum**), fractures of the ossicular chain creating a discontinuity, or a TM perforation. Hearing assessment and subsequent treatment can be done after the acute, more serious injuries have been stabilized.

Eye Care in Facial Paralysis:

The facial nerve provides a critical function to the eye, namely, eyelid closure. This action provides a valuable protective function of maintaining moisture to the **cornea** over the external surface. The eyelid blink sweeps tears over the cornea, and eyelid closure at night prevents the cornea from drying. Without this protection, the cornea can become progressively more dry, causing significant pain, **corneal ulceration**, scarring, and ultimately permanent changes in vision. In addition, the eyelid blink reflex protects the eye by preventing foreign bodies from contacting the surface and damaging the cornea. Patients with facial nerve paralysis need to use artificial tears frequently during the day, as well as a moisture lubricant at night while they sleep. They may also wear a clear plastic moisture chamber for protection and humidification. The best treatment for corneal injuries is prevention by early use of lubricating drops and moisturizing lubricants and chambers.

Surgical rehabilitation is possible with placement of a gold weight into the upper eye lid. This allows gravity to pull the eyelid down. An almost natural appearance and function results.

Questions, Section #8

1. Peripheral facial paralysis can be due to _____,
    _____, _____, or
    _____.

2. Facial paralysis without an identified etiology is termed
    _____.

3. Bell's palsy is commonly due to _____ and
    should be treated with _____ and
    _____.

Answers

1. TUMORS OF PAROTID OR SKULL BASE, INFECTIONS,
    TRAUMA, CHOLESTEATOMA
2. BELL'S PALSY
3. VIRAL OR HERPETIC INFECTION, STEROIDS,
    ANTIVIRALS

Patients present to the primary care practitioners with a variety of nasal complaints, ranging from **rhinorrhea** and **postnasal drainage** to obstruction and pain. Rhinorrhea and post nasal drainage can result from allergic rhinitis, nonallergic rhinitis (the patient tests negative for allergies) vasomotor rhinitis (typically worsens with eating, change in temperature, or bright light) and acute and chronic rhinosinusitis. Nasal obstruction can be caused by anatomic deformities such as **septal and external nasal deviation, turbinate hypertrophy,** nasal polyps, and inflammatory changes resulting in **mucosal edema.**

Successful treatment of the varying causes of rhinorrhea and obstruction is based on an accurate diagnosis of the underlying cause. Allergic rhinitis and viral rhinosinusitis are the 2 most common nasal problems encountered. Allergic rhinitis can be differentiated from acute viral respiratory infection by history and physical examination. Patients with allergic rhinitis have a history of **atopy**, sneezing, watery eyes, possible **seasonal predilection**, and prolonged symptoms in comparison to patients with viral disease. Allergic patients have congested, pale nasal mucosa with clear drainage and are afebrile.

The 2nd-generation **antihistamines** such as cetirizine, fexofenadine, or loratadine are very well tolerated and effective in allergic rhinitis. Decongestants taken alone or in combination with antihistamines taken orally will help many patients with drainage and congestion. They are often helpful to people who have symptoms for only several weeks out of the year. Patients who have symptoms for longer periods generally do better on one of the **intranasal steroid sprays**. Topical intranasal steroid sprays are considered the first line of treatment for allergic rhinitis. Note they do not reach their full effectiveness until 6 continuous weeks of therapy, and patients should take them for 6 weeks before deciding whether they are working. Cromolyn sodium and azelastine sprays are also available as treatment for allergic rhinitis. If your patients don't respond to these treatments, **specific desensitization therapy (allergy shots)** is indicated. These patients sometimes have very large turbinates and can benefit from **surgical reduction of the intranasal structures**. Vasomotor rhinitis and nonallergic rhinitis can **mimic** allergic rhinitis. In both, patients present with clear rhinorrhea and no other allergic symptoms or history. The allergy tests are negative. Vasomotor rhinitis is often triggered by eating, temperature change, or sudden bright light. Intranasal steroid sprays are the best treatment for non-allergic and vasomotor rhinitis.

The "Common Cold":

Acute viral rhinosinusitis is frequently attributed to one of a multitude of rhinoviruses and results in symptoms we refer to as the "common cold." The pathophysiology involves infection, inflammation, mucosal swelling, and increased mucus production. Low-grade fever, facial discomfort, and purulent nasal drainage are commonly encountered. Treatment is symptomatic. Treatment of symptoms with antipyretics, hydration, analgesics, and decongestants recommended, as needed. Spontaneous resolution occurs in 7-10 days.

50

Antibiotic treatment of the common cold is discouraged. Unfortunately, patients often request (demand) antibiotics early in the course of viral illness. When spontaneous recovery occurs, they assume that the antibiotics were responsible. This is a major cause of excessive antibiotic use and has contributed to the surge in antibiotic resistance.

Acute Bacterial Rhinosinusitis:

Prolonged mucosal edema from whatever etiology causes sinus obstruction and retention of secretions and may lead to **acute bacterial rhinosinusitis**. Patients may

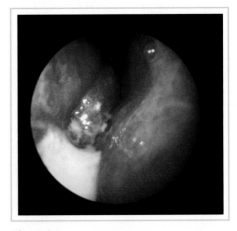

Figure 9.1.

Acute rhinosinusitis. Note purulent drainage extending from the middle meatus over the inferior turbinate. Symptoms persisting longer than 7-10 days suggest bacterial infection, and antibiotic therapy is indicated.

exhibit several of the major symptoms (facial pressure, pain, prulent discharge, nasal obstruction, anosmia, headache) and one or more of the minor symptoms (fever, cough, toothache, halitosis). **Radiographic studies** (plain films, computed tomography [CT] scans) do not differentiate acute bacterial rhinosinusitis from a viral upper respiratory infection (URI). More than 80% of patients with a viral URI have an abnormal sinus CT scan. Time will usually differentiate a bacterial from viral infection. It usually takes 7-10 days for a viral infection to resolve. Symptoms lasting beyond 7-10 days, or worsening after 5 days, suggest that bacterial infection is being established. The organisms that cause this are similar to the organisms that cause acute otitis media and include *Streptococcus pneumoniae, Haemophilus influenzae*, and *Moraxella catarrhalis*. By definition, acute rhinosinusitis persists up to 30 days. **Subacute rhinosinusitis** lasts up to 3 months, and sinusitis that persists past 3 months is termed **chronic sinusitis** and usually has a different microbiology, with increased numbers of anaerobic organisms.

The treatment of choice for acute rhinosinusitis (as well as acute otitis media) has been either amoxicillin or trimethoprim/sulfamethoxazole for 10 days. Resistance to amoxicillin has prompted some physicians to consider using amoxicillin/clavulanate or a 2nd-generation cephalosporin or macrolide or a quinolone instead of amoxicillin as the first-line therapy. More recently, the appearance of penicillin resistance in *S. pneumoniae* infection (which has a different resistance mechanism than beta-lactamase production) has resulted in the recommendation that higher doses of amoxicillin be used routinely. In uncomplicated rhinosinusitis, no current data suggest that 2nd or 3rd generation drugs are superior to amoxicillin or folate inhibitors. In complicated cases, recurrent sinusitis, or failure of initial treatment, however, they may be of value. Drugs that do not adequately cover *H. influenzae* are inappropriate treatment for otitis media and rhinosinusitis.

In addition to antibiotic therapy many adjunctive measures may include topical decongestants (oxymetazoline) for 3 days, mucolytics (guaifenisen) and oral decongestants. Severe or recurrent cases may require systemic steroids. Antihistamines and topical steroids are not particularly indicated unless allergy is also a major concern.

Patients with sinusitis should be **referred** to an otolaryngologist if they have **3-4 infections per year, an infection that does not respond to**

51

two three-week courses of antibiotics, nasal polyps, or complication of sinusitis including those described below.

Several types of acute sinusitis merit further mention. Acute frontal, ethmoid, and sphenoid sinusitis that aren't appropriately treated or don't respond to therapy can have serious consequences.

Frontal Sinusitis:

The frontal sinus lining has veins that penetrate the posterior sinus wall and go directly to the dura on the opposite side. These veins can quite easily **transmit organisms** or become **pathways for propagation of an infected clot**. This can lead quickly to meningitis and even brain abscess, in fact, the most common cause of frontal lobe abscess is frontal sinusitis. Therefore, the diagnosis of acute frontal sinusitis with an **air-fluid level** requires **aggressive** antibiotic therapy. The key to frontal sinusitis is to cover *S. pneumoniae*, and *H. influenzae* as well as get good cerebrospinal fluid penetration.

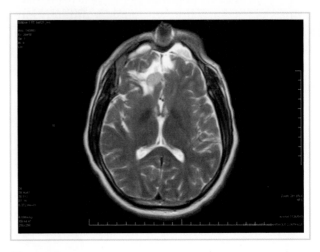

Figure 9.2.

This axial CT scan depicts a patient with fluid in his right frontal sinus. The infection has spread retrograde and he has developed a frontal abscess.

Pain is severe, and patients usually require admission for treatment and close observation. **Topical vasoconstriction** to shrink the swollen mucosa around the nasofrontal duct and restore natural drainage into the nose is begun in the clinic and used often throughout the hospital stay. Systemic steroids may also be considered to decrease swelling. If frontal sinusitis doesn't greatly improve within 24 hours, the frontal sinus should be surgically drained to prevent serious **intracranial infections**.

Ethmoid Sinusitis:

Severe ethmoid sinusitis can result in **orbital cellulitis** or abscess. These patients present with **eyelid swelling, proptosis,** and **double vision.** However, the double vision, instead of being due to the involvement of the nerves of the cavernous sinus, may be due to an abscess located in the orbit. A CT scan will generally show the presence (or absence) of an abscess, which is always accompanied by ethmoid sinusitis. If an abscess is present, it will require surgical drainage as soon as possible. However, if the condition is severe ethmoid sinusitis without abscess, it may be treated with intravenous antibiotics and nasal flushes with decongestant nose drops. If the patient's condition worsens, then surgery is indicated. However, severe ethmoid sinusitis will often resolve with nonoperative therapy.

Sphenoid Sinusitis:

Sphenoid sinusitis can cause **ophthalmoplegia,** meningitis, and even **cavernous sinus thrombosis.** Cavernous sinus thrombosis is a complication with even more grave implications than meningitis or brain abscess, and it carries a mortality of approximately 50%. The veins of the face that drain the sinuses don't have valves, and they may drain posteriorly into the cavernous sinus. **Infectious venous thrombophlebitis** can spread into the cavernous sinus from a source on the face or in the sinus. The most common cause of this serious infection is rhinosinusitis.

The nerves that run through the cavernous sinus are the oculomotor (III), trochlear (IV), and 1st and 2nd divisions of the trigeminal (V) and the abducens (VI). A patient who has double vision and rhinosinusitis may be thought to have cavernous sinus thrombosis until it is ruled out. The treatment is high-dose intravenous antibiotics and surgical drainage of the **paranasal sinuses.** Anticoagulation is also a consideration in the treatment regimen. CT and/or MRI scans are necessary to diagnose cavernous sinus thrombosis.

Nasal Obstruction:

Nasal obstruction is another common nasal complaint seen regularly in the ENT office setting. A frequent cause of nasal obstruction is **septal deviation.** These patients often present with histories of nasal obstruction, possibly complicated by sinusitis and headaches. They may also snore and have obstructive sleep apnea syndrome. Surgery readily corrects the nasal obstruction and can reduce chronic sinusitis and headaches. Studies have shown that correction of the nasal obstruction rarely cures the sleep apnea. When the obstruction involves the nasal pyramid, it, too, must be corrected by **rhinoplasty**. Rhinoplasty involves controlled chisel cuts of the bones (**osteotomies**) on either side of the nose and placement of the bones into the correct position. (Rhinoplasty can be combined with trimming of the nasal cartilage to subtly change the contour of the tip of the nose.) This is held in place with a splint for a week after surgery.

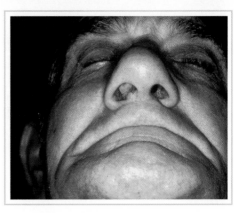

Figure 9.3.

View of nose of a patient with a deviated nasal septum. Note that the cartilaginous septum extends into the right nostril, resulting in impaired airflow. Most septal deviations are not as dramatic as this and can be visualized only with rhinoscopy.

54

Nasal Polyps:

Nasal polyps are localized, extremely edematous nasal or sinus mucosa. Microscopically they are essentially full of water. They can enlarge while in the nose and obstruct either the nose or the ostia through which the sinuses drain. The exact cause of polyps is not known, but fifty percent of patients who have polyps also have allergies, so patients with polyps are evaluated for allergies.

Polyps usually respond very well to a course of systemic steroids followed by continuous intranasal steroid sprays. If they do not respond or reoccur frequently then surgery may be indicated.

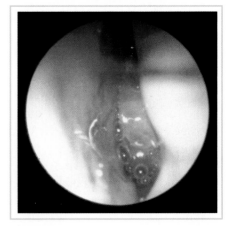

Figure 9.4.

Photograph of a nasal polyp. Nasal polyposis is a common ailment that results in nasal obstruction and drainage. Most patients require medical treatment with topical steroids and antibiotics as well as surgical removal of polyps and diseased tissue.

Unilateral nasal polyps may be a manifestation of a **neoplasm,** and must be referred to an otolaryngologist for evaluation. Nasal polyps are also a frequent cause of nasal blockage. Patients with allergic rhinitis and chronic sinusitis develop these grapelike swellings that protrude into the **lumen**, causing obstruction and **anosmia**. These polyps are often associated with **asthma**. Medical therapy with inhaled nasal steroids as well as short bursts of systemic steroids often produces good long-term control of the disease. Surgical removal provides relief, but, unfortunately, recurrence is common. **Triad** asthma (Samter's triad), which involves asthma, aspirin allergy, and nasal polyposis, is a particularly difficult form of this disease.

Another relatively frequent cause of nasal blockage is **rhinitis medica-mentosa**. This syndrome develops when people repeatedly use decongestant nasal sprays over a long period. The rebound effect causes them to need the spray just to breathe. After prolonged use, the mucosa becomes quite inflamed. The treatment is discontinuation of the decongestant sprays. Symptoms can be reduced by the use of an intranasal steroid spray, occasionally accompanied by short bursts of systemic steroids. Cocaine abuse can also cause this problem. Cocaine may also induce **ischemic necrosis in the nasal septum** because of the amount of vaso-constriction. The ischemia then may result in a **nasal septal perforation**, which interferes with nasal airflow and is very difficult to repair surgically.

In addition, some patients have a very straight septum with no nasal polyposis or inflammation, but they suffer from chronic rhinosinusitis due to blockage of sinus drainage. The **uncinate process** comes very close to the **ethmoid bulla**, forming the **infundibulum** through which the **maxillary sinus** drains. Only 1 mm of swelling in the mucosa in this area will obstruct the sinus **ostium**. Patients with chronic obstruction in this area and recurrent sinusitis often undergo surgery to remove the uncinate process and open the bulla to let the ethmoid and maxillary sinuses drain more freely. After the surgery, a small amount of swelling won't obstruct the drainage flow from these sinuses. This procedure is now done endoscopically, and patients tolerate it very well.

Nasal Masses:

By far the most common nasal mass encountered by physicians are nasal polyps. As expected they present with symptoms that are due to the obstruction caused by the mass being present. Obstruction of the natural osteum of the sinus will cause a backup and may lead to sinusitis.

Questions, Section #9

1. A patient complains of fatigue, low grade fever, purulent rhinorrhea, and headache that resolves within 7 days. The most likely diagnosis is a _____.

2. A patient had a typical cold that did not resolve in 10 days and now has fatigue, purulent rhinorrhea, low-grade fever, and headache for 3 weeks. The most likely diagnosis is _____.

3. Another patient has similar symptoms for more than 3 months. This patient has _____.

4. A common cause of nasal obstruction that is easily corrected by surgery is a _____.

5. Triad asthma (Samter's triad) consists of asthma, nasal polyposis, and _____.

6. Unilateral nasal polyps can either be caused by or be a manifestation of a _____and therefore warrant referral to an otolaryngologist.

7. Any patient with symptoms of sinusitis and _____ should be referred to an otolaryngologist immediately.

8. Patients should see an otolaryngologist if they have_____ episodes of sinusitis per year or if they have any_____ of sinusitis.

Answers

1. COLD
2. ACUTE RHINOSINUSITIS
3. CHRONIC RHINOSINUSITIS
4. DEVIATED SEPTUM
5. ASPIRIN ALLERGY
6. NEOPLASM
7. DOUBLE VISION
8. 3-4, COMPLICATION

The important thing in science is not so much to obtain new facts, as to discover new ways of thinking about them.

Sir William Bragg

The standard radiographic study for evaluation of sinus disease is the sinus CT scan performed in the **coronal plane** without intravenous contrast. As in other radiographic studies, a few principles go a long way.

- The 1st thing you look at is the **name**.
- The 2nd thing you look at is the **date**.
- The 3rd thing you look at is the **orientation— right versus left**.

The convention of designating sides for head and neck CT scans varies from institution to institution. You **can't assume** that if the film is positioned so you can read the name, that right is right and left is left. You <u>must</u> see an *R* or an *L*.

There are **4 radiographic densities: air, fat, water, and bone**.

Remember this very basic principle: When 2 structures of the same radiographic density are adjacent, the border between them is obscured. For example, if you can't see the right heart border on a **posterior-anterior (PA)** chest x-ray, the lung next to the heart (right middle lobe) has the same density (water density) as the heart. Likewise, pus or fluid in the sinus has the same density as thickening of the sinus mucosa.

The relative density of bone and other structures can be manipulated by the radiologist during viewing of the scan and printed, typically as either bone window (demonstrates clear bone detail) or soft tissue window (bones too bright, soft tissue easily visualized).

When you view CT scans, you must look at more than one image. If you don't know what a structure is, follow it through adjacent slices and you will usually be able to easily identify the anatomic structure that you are viewing.

Using a **systematic** way to review any imaging study in sequence is critical to avoid missing subtle abnormalities. Although the novice viewer routinely examines the maxillary sinuses first, you should systematically evaluate the orbits, orbital walls, **maxillary alveolus,** nasal septum, and sinuses. Remember that the ethmoid sinuses lie between the orbits, the maxillary sinus below the orbits, frontal above, and sphenoid behind. **You should carefully study every x-ray, MRI, or CT scan that you encounter,** so you can learn to recognize common anatomic variants and distinguish them from true pathology.

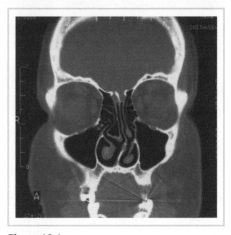

Figure 10.1.

CT scan of patient with deviated nasal septum and an ethmoid air cell within the middle turbinate. The surgical correction of nasal obstruction in this patient would require partial middle turbinectomy as well as correction of the deviated nasal septum.

Here are 3 common anatomic variants encountered on coronal CT scans of the sinuses. See figures 10.1 to 10.3.

58

1. Deviated nasal septum

2. Asymmetry of sinuses, including size, shape, presence of septas, etc.

3. An air cell within the middle turbinate (**concha bullosa)**

Abnormalities include fluid, mucosal thickening, bony fractures, cysts, and tumors. Look for these in figures 10.1 to 10.3.

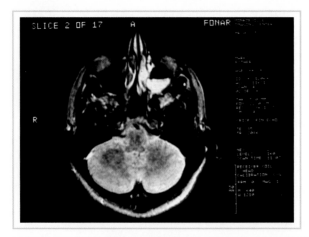

Figure 10.2.

Axial MRI scan of a patient with an air fluid level in his left maxillary sinus. A coronal CT scan is the preferred study for the evaluation of sinusitis; however, disease can also be readily seen on axial CT scans, often obtained for other reasons.

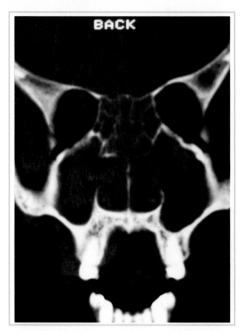

BACK

Figure 10.3.

Pansinusitis with polyps, mucosal edema (or fluid-filling nose), ethmoid sinus, and maxillary sinuses.

The Osteomeatal Complex:

The most significant area to examine in a patient with sinus complaints is the **osteomeatal complex (OMC)**. Coronal CT scans are used in the evaluation of sinus disease because they are best for visualizing the OMC. (However, axial CT scans are better for evaluation of the frontal sinuses). The OMC is the region through which the maxillary sinus drains in the nose. Edema obstructing the OMC will frequently lead to chronic maxillary sinusitis. This edema can be minimal, and is usually associated with clouding of the anterior ethmoid sinuses. The most anterior ethmoid sinus—the **agger nasi cell**—is frequently clouded. Edema in this sinus may be associated with obstruction of the nasal frontal duct, which isn't well visualized on a CT scan, and results in frontal sinusitis.

In most instances, sinusitis is manifested by loss of aeration of multiple sinuses, usually involving both sides. This is water density, which may be swelling of the mucosa or polyps, fluid, or pus. Clouding of a single sinus (unilateral disease) is unusual and suggests an unusual cause, such as a tumor.

A sinus CT scan is not the first step in the evaluation of a patient with chronic sinusitis. Moreover, it is not necessary in the evaluation of all patients since the history and physical, particularly nasal endoscopy, will often identify the source of the pathology. Medical therapy, consisting of antibiotics, decongestants and topical steroids can be initiated based on clinical criteria. Should the patient fail this, or experience multiple episodes of sinusitis, then a sinus CT is essential for determining if there is an anatomic cause for the problem. If surgical intervention is

59

being considered, then the CT scan provides valuable information, that is essential to the pre-operative plan.

It should be noted that all patients with nasal polyposis have chronic sinusitis, typically involving all sinuses. Unilateral nasal polyposis associated with unilateral sinusitis suggests tumor (most commonly, **inverted papilloma,** a benign growth caused by human papilloma virus [HPV]).

Mucosal thickening of the sinuses, particularly, the ethmoid sinuses, persists 6-8 weeks following a URI. Each of us can expect to suffer 3 or 4 URIs per year, so random sinus CT scans performed on a population will demonstrate a high incidence of mucosal thickening. As a result, it's important that the CT scan be obtained after a patient has been maximally treated, and the disease is at its nadir or most improved state. On a CT scan it's impossible to differentiate between sinus clouding due to a common cold or due to bacterial sinusitis.

Remember: The best way to learn to look at any x-ray or imaging study is to carefully and systematically examine as many as possible.

Questions, Section #10

1. The 1st thing you should look at on any x-ray or CT scan is
   _____.

2. The 2nd thing you should look at on any x-ray is
   _____.

3. The 3rd thing you should look at on any x-ray (and especially on a CT scan) is _____.

4. The 4 radiographic densities are _____, _____, _____, and _____.

5. When 2 structures of the same radiographic density are adjacent to each other, the border between them becomes _____.

6. CT scans are typically printed in 1 of 2 densities, _____ density and _____ density.

7. CT scans are typically obtained in the coronal plane because this view best demonstrates the _____.

8. Common anatomic variants encountered on coronal CT scans include _____, _____, _____.

9. The key area that must be visualized on a sinus CT scan is the
   _____.

10. The best way to learn to look at an x-ray or other imaging study is to carefully examine _____ in a systematic fashion.

Answers

1. THE NAME
2. THE DATE
3. IDENTIFICATION OF RIGHT AND LEFT SIDE
4. AIR, FAT, WATER, BONE
5. OBSCURED
6. BONE, SOFT TISSUE
7. OSTEOMEATAL COMPLEX (OMC)
8. ASYMMETRIES OF SINUSES, DEVIATED SEPTUM, CONCHA BULLOSA
9. OSTEOMEATAL COMPLEX (OMC)
10. AS MANY AS POSSIBLE

Nothing in this world can take the place of persistence. Talent will not; nothing is more common than unsuccessful men with talent. Genius will not; unrewarded genius is almost a proverb. Education will not; the world is full of educated derelicts. Persistence and determination alone are omnipotent.

Calvin Coolidge

When you are treating maxillofacial trauma, obviously, the basic (ABC) tenets of trauma management hold:

1. You must secure an **A**irway.

2. You must make sure the patient is **B**reathing and ventilating adequately.

3. You must ensure adequate **C**irculation by stopping bleeding and providing fluid replacement.

4. You must ensure that no **C**-spine fracture is present.

First, the airway. Health care professionals always wonder whether a patient should have a cricothyrotomy or intubation. This is, indeed, sometimes a judgment call. One way of thinking about this is to go down a checklist of ways to secure the airway.

Don't forget that the most common cause of airway obstruction in a patient with an altered level of consciousness is the tongue falling back into the throat. This can be treated by a **jaw lift maneuver**, an **oral airway**, or a **long nasal airway**. Don't forget the possibility of a foreign body (dentures in adults; balloons, small toys, food, etc., in children) obstructing the airway. If the cause of airway obstruction isn't so simple, however, the quickest and easiest method of securing the airway is **endotracheal intubation** through the mouth. This requires placing a laryngoscope down through the mouth to the larynx (**direct laryngoscopy**) and lifting up. The **vocal cords** are seen and then the tube is placed into the trachea. But this technique may not work for two reasons. The first reason is if the patient has a broken neck. Direct laryngoscopy requires movement of the neck, and if the neck is broken, it can possibly move during the procedure and compress the spinal cord, causing paraplegia, quadriplegia, or death. Therefore, oral endotracheal intubation is not to be performed if a patient has either a known C-spine fracture or the possibility of having a C-spine fracture that hasn't been ruled out by a lateral neck film. The second

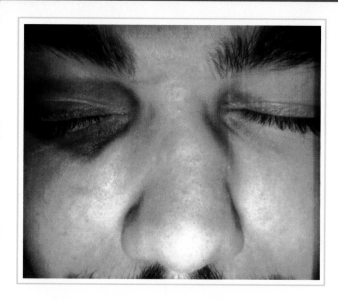

Figure 11.1.

Nasal fracture. Note that the bony nasal pyramid has been shifted toward the patients left. This is the most common direction because patients who suffer from this injury are most likely to have been struck by a right-handed individual! Repair is straightforward but should be completed within 5-7 days to ensure optimal outcome.

reason you might not be able to perform oral intubation is massive trauma with distortion of landmarks and bleeding. The patient might actually have had a lateral C-spine film that showed no C-spine fracture; however, at direct laryngoscopy, all you can see is blood and torn tissue. This patient will obviously need a surgical airway. You would perform a cricothyrotomy unless there is concern over a **fractured larynx (widened thyroid cartilage, subcutaneous air [crepitus], neck bruising, hoarseness, coughing up blood)**, in which case, a tracheotomy is the procedure of choice. Remember: Normal lateral C-spine film doesn't completely rule out a C-spine fracture. Intubation in a trauma situation requires that **in-line cervical traction** be applied to the head by someone other than the intubating doctor at the time of intubation.

Next on the checklist, if you can't perform an oral intubation, you can sometimes perform a **fiberoptic nasotracheal intubation.** In this case, an endotracheal tube is passed through the nose down into the **hypopharynx,** guided by a fiberoptic endoscope placed through the endotracheal tube. With the endoscope, you can see when the tube approaches the larynx, and immediately after an expiration, the scope is advanced into the larynx. You must wait until just after an expiration because the vocal cords open when the patient takes a breath in, and this is an ideal time to push the endoscope through. Once the endo-scope is in the trachea, the tube is passed over it and the endoscope is

63

removed. The advantage of the fiberoptic nasotracheal intubation technique is that the neck isn't manipulated at all, so if a C-spine fracture hasn't been ruled out, it is still a viable option. However, this technique isn't feasible if visualization is obscured by secretions, blood, or swelling. Also, if there is a **severe midface injury** with possible **cribriform plate fracture,** then passage of a nasogastric or blind nasotracheal tube is contraindicated because the tube may pass into the brain.

You now come to the 3rd option in airway management. You've gone through your checklist as above and determined that the patient's tongue isn't the problem, you can't perform an oral intubation (perhaps because the lateral C-spine film shows a broken neck), and you can't perform a nasotracheal intubation (perhaps because the patient has profuse oral bleeding). You then realize that the only option is a surgical airway. The

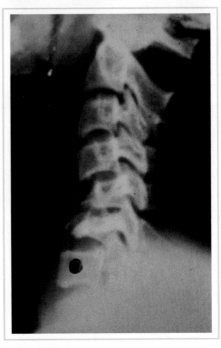

Figure 11.2.

Lateral C-spine x-ray of a patient who suffered a facial injury. The black dot marks vertebra C7. Care must be taken to ensure that all 7 cervical vertebrae are visible. Head and neck stabilization is required in all serious head and neck injuries until there is radiographic evidence that the C-spine is uninjured.

method of choice is a tracheotomy or a cricothyrotomy. In an emergency, cricothyrotomy may be chosen over tracheotomy because it's quicker and is accomplished through the relatively thin cricothyroid membrane. You should learn to palpate and recognize the cricoid cartilage. Try it on yourself. The membrane is just above the cricoid cartilage, below the thyroid cartilage (the Adam's apple). The choice of which procedure to perform may depend on the level of expertise available.

Other Aspects of Maxillofacial Trauma Management:

Any person who has sustained enough trauma to break a facial bone should be assumed to have a C-spine fracture until this is ruled out. Rule

#1 in maxillofacial trauma management is secure the **A**irway, **B**reathing, and **C**irculation. Rule #2 is rule out a C-spine fracture if it hasn't already been done. Rule #3 is evaluate the patient completely. Look in the ears for hemotympanum, which can signify a temporal bone fracture. Check that the facial nerve works on both sides, since a complication of temporal bone fracture may be facial nerve paralysis. Any temporal bone fracture is something for which an otolaryngologist should be consulted. Next, palpate the orbital rims to ascertain whether or not a **malar (tripod) fracture** has occurred. Make sure the patient isn't experiencing double vision, which can occur when an **orbital blowout fracture** happens and the **inferior rectus** or **medial rectus** can become entrapped. Make sure that there is no **infraorbital nerve hypesthesia,** which can also occur with a blowout fracture or a tripod fracture.

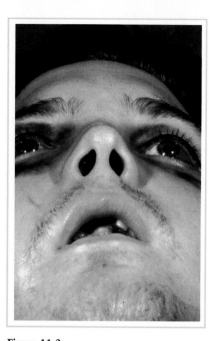

Figure 11.3.

Bilateral periorbital ecchymoses and sub-conjunctival hemorrhages. This may be due to soft tissue trauma only, or it may be a manifestation of underlying fracture.

65

Next, evaluate the nose. In general, isolated nasal fractures can be reduced up to 14 days after the fracture, if they cause a cosmetic deformity or airway obstruction. It is easier to do when there is less swelling and, usually, the swelling goes down by 5-7 days. If the septum has been broken, you must rule out a **septal hematoma**, the formation of a blood clot between the **perichondrium** and cartilage that disrupts the nourishment of the cartilage. This can result in **septal necrosis,** with subsequent perforation due to either a loss of nutrition from the perichondrium or a secondary infection of the hematoma, generally with *Staphylococcus aureus*. These are treated by incision and drainage and packing to ensure that they don't re-accumulate. Remember: Radiographs aren't particularly helpful in cases of a broken nose, because old fractures can't be distinguished from acute ones. Generally, inspection and palpation are the best ways to diagnose a broken nose. Uncomplicated nasal fractures are treated with antibiotics, pain medicine, a decongestant nasal spray, and a referral for reduction within 3-5 days.

Continuing with the exam, evaluate the stability of the maxilla by grasping the maxilla area just above the front teeth and applying a gentle rocking motion. If the maxilla is unstable, you will feel it move separately from the face. This is a **LeFort fracture**

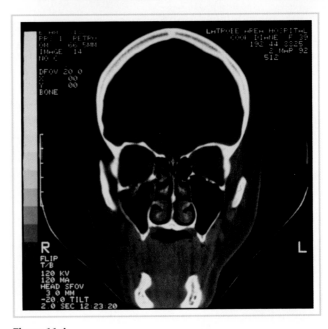

Figure 11.4.

Coronal CT scan demonstrating a blowout fracture of the right orbit. This fracture often results in entrapment of the inferior rectus muscle and limitation of upward gaze.

and will require **surgical plating**. A complete bilateral LeFort III fracture is rare and involves massive trauma, usually with spinal fluid leakage. The procedure involves disarticulating the face from the skull. The remaining soft tissue attachments consist largely of the optic nerves, thus the *gentle* rocking. A CT scan will elucidate the situation if you are unsure.

Check the patient for **cerebrospinal fluid (CSF)** rhinorrhea, since a basal skull fracture or temporal bone fracture can leak first into the middle ear, which drains down into the Eustachian tube and out the nose. Alternatively, the site of leak may be just above the cribriform plate. Remember that CSF mixed with blood produces a ring sign on the sheets or on filter paper and also that CSF has a measurable glucose concentration, and mere nasal secretions do not. Beta-transferrin is a protein only found in CSF. So a positive test is diagnostic of a CSF leak.

Evaluate the mandible. Examine the patient's occlusion and ask if his or her teeth fit together like they always have. Mandibular fractures are generally treated with a combination of intermaxillary fixation and the surgical application of plates.

Trauma to the neck may injure the larynx or trachea. For example, blunt trauma from a steering wheel or garrote can cause fracture of the thyroid cartilage, cricoid, or both. A complete crush isn't compatible with life unless someone handy with a knife is waiting to do an immediate cricothyrotomy— lesser injury generally results in progressive hoarseness and **stridor**. The only initial physical finding may be **cervical ecchymosis**. Check for loss of cartilaginous landmarks and feel for subcutaneous air (**subcutaneous emphysema**). Any positive finding is an indication for further evaluation with laryngoscopy, possible CT, and observation. Penetrating wounds to the neck may also indicate injury to the vascular structures or airway. Immediate expert evaluation will determine if surgery is required.

Questions, Section #11

1. The first priority in management of maxillofacial trauma is securing the_____.

2. In an unconscious patient, the most common cause of airway obstruction is _____.

3. Two reasons that oral endotracheal intubation may be contraindicated are _____ and _____.

4. A contraindication to blind nasotracheal or nasogastric intubation is _____.

5. The nerve that is commonly not evaluated upon initial presentation, but whose management depends greatly on the examination at the initial time of presentation is the _____ nerve.

6. A fractured nose can be reduced in up to 14 days without complications; however, a _____ must be ruled out at the time of the initial fracture.

Answers

1. AIRWAY
2. PROLAPSE OF THE TONGUE POSTERIORLY
3. A BROKEN NECK, MASSIVE TRAUMA WITH DISTORTION OF LANDMARKS AND BLEEDING
4. CRIBRIFORM PLATE FRACTURE
5. FACIAL
6. SEPTAL HEMATOMA

A large part of otolaryngology involves performance of facial plastic surgery. This runs the gamut from doing **traumatic repairs** on lacerations of the face to **reconstruction** after cancer, and then to purely **cosmetic** procedures such as a facelift (**rhytidectomy**). Here are some of the basic principles involved in taking care of patients with injuries or deformities of the face.

Soft Tissue Trauma:

It is often very striking when patients present after suffering massive facial trauma. They may have large flaps of tissue that have been folded back, exposing the underlying

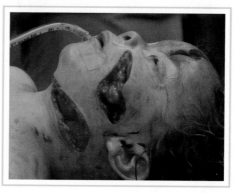

Figure 12.1.

This patient was an unrestrained passenger in a motor vehicle accident. They have multiple facial lacerations, contusions and fractures. Remember the ABC's in their management.

anatomy. They may also have some areas of tissue that are missing. Facial disfigurement from fractured and displaced facial bones, may be present. Often, there is blood, mud, and maybe even a little beer in the wound. These patients have an "Oh, wow!" effect when you see them for the workup. The workup should begin with the basics of trauma management: **evaluation of all other associated injuries**, administration of **antibiotics,** and a **tetanus shot,** if needed. Don't forget to check to be sure that the C-spine has been cleared. Smaller lacerations can be taken care of satisfactorily in the emergency room. Sometimes, however, it's best to go to the operating room, especially if repair will require more than an hour or so. Once you are down to managing these soft tissue injuries of the face, a few principles will help.

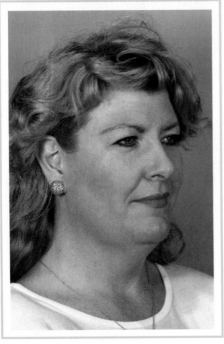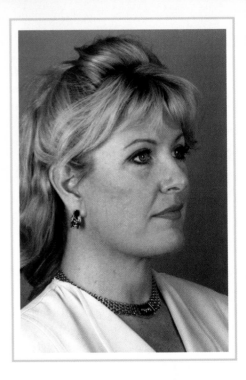

70 **Figure 12.2(a, b).**

Pre- and postop photographs of a woman who has undergone facial rejuvenation. She has had surgery to her eyelids (blepharoplasties), removal of fat from her neck (liposuction), and resection of excessive facial skin (facelift). Improvement in facial appearance is often dramatic (as in this case) and secondary benefits through enhancement of self-esteem may be even more dramatic.

The first principle is careful reapproximation of all remaining tissue. After the wound has been anesthetized and cleansed, it becomes obvious where the tissues need to go. It is important to be meticulous when you are reapproximating them, somewhat like putting together a jigsaw puzzle! Line up known lines first: rather as in a split-image viewfinder on a 35-mm camera, the vermilion border of the lips, **free margins of the nasal filtrum** (the line from the bottom of the nose to the upper lip), and edges of eyebrows, eyelids, and parts of the pinna must be perfectly aligned. If you don't get them right the first time, cut out the sutures and do it again. Deep sutures of **polyglactin** help to reduce the tension placed on the actual skin wound. Take care to evert the wound edges as much as possible, especially when placing the skin stitches. Nylon or polypropylene is usually used on the skin. On the face, 5-0 or

6-0 suture is usually adequate. Immediately after a wound is closed, it fills with serum, which clots. This serum prevents water from entering the wound. Please don't make a patient keep a wound dry for a week—a wound may be allowed to get wet within a few minutes of closure if the microscopic clot isn't disrupted. Thus, you may tell patients they can get their wound wet as long as they don't scrub it. Do ask them to keep ointment on a wound, to retain moisture and reduce crusting until the skin has grown across (usually about a week on the face).

Skin stitches on the face should be removed at 3-5 days, and allowed to remain somewhat longer on the ear and scalp, usually around 7 days. It is important for patients to realize that scars take a minimum of 1 year to mature because a complex biologic process goes on in the formation of a scar. The time course usually involves the scar turning very red, with the maximum redness occurring at approximately 6 weeks. It then tends to fade to purple and brown before eventually turning white. In general, scar revisions aren't done until a scar has matured for at least a year. Sunscreen should be used for at least the 1st year after the injury because scars can become **hyperpigmented** with exposure to the sun. Occasionally, if **hypertrophic** scars tend to form, steroid injections into them can help. Recently, early **dermabrasion** (like sanding a piece of wood), at 6-8 weeks, has been used with success in reducing scarring. Timing of this procedure is critical. Covering the wound with silastic sheeting, has recently been shown to decrease exuberent scars.

Septorhinoplasty:

Perhaps the most common form of facial plastic surgery that an oto-laryngologist performs is a **septorhinoplasty**. In this operation, the deviated septum is straightened and the outside of the nose may also be changed in form through various surgical maneuvers. The most common procedure is straightening the septum (**septoplasty**), which is performed through the nostrils and entails realignment of the septum into the midline.

Changing the external contour of the nose is called **rhinoplasty**. The most important part of rhinoplasty is maintaining or improving the airway, so a septoplasty is usually performed as part of this procedure. Patients who can't breathe through their nose after an operation will be very dissatisfied because it takes much more physiologic work to breathe through the mouth than it does through the nose.

Classically, rhinoplasty was performed on people with large dorsal humps. However, patients' sophistication and demands have changed. We now find ourselves restructuring and recontouring the outside of the nose, often even augmenting it instead of making it smaller. Anyone's most attractive feature is the eyes, so the end cosmetic goal of rhinoplasty is to keep the nose from drawing attention away from the eyes. Over-reduction of the bony and cartilaginous framework of the nose leads to long-term cosmetic deformity and, often, airway compromise. Surgical correction of this **iatrogenic** problem is challenging at best, and tends to be unrewarding for both the patient and the surgeon.

Blepharoplasty:

Blepharoplasty is often performed by otolaryngologists who perform facial plastic surgery. When the upper lid skin becomes redundant dermatochalasia, they can actually obstruct the upper field of vision. When this is the case, the skin can be removed to allow better vision. This is the main functional benefit of a blepharoplasty; however, patients also will often desire some cosmetic changes around their eyes. Bulges that occur below the eyes consist of orbital fat pressing against a weakened orbital septum. This fat can be resected, along with extra skin and muscle. However, this must be done with great care, as there is little margin for error, especially around the lower lid.

Other Facial Plastic Surgery:

Occasionally, the eyebrows lie below the level of the superior orbital rim. This is called brow **ptosis** and can cause an apparent excess of skin in the upper lid. Elevation of the brow with a brow lift can reduce redundant skin of the eyelids.

A natural extension of a brow lift includes surgery for the rest of the aging face. This can include a forehead lift, a facelift, **chemical peeling, laser resurfacing,** and dermabrasion. A facelift removes slack facial skin and is performed through incisions that run in front of the ear, up into the scalp, and behind the ear into the scalp. The operation involves undermining the skin over the face and neck, with resuspending of the platysma muscle, cheek fat pad, and, in some cases, the **orbicularis oculi** muscle. The skin is then redraped and the excess skin trimmed. Occasionally, very fine wrinkles aren't addressed by this procedure, so patients will choose either a chemical peel, dermabrasion, or laser resurfacing. This is usually necessary, especially around the mouth, where **perioral rhytids** tend to be very prominent.

Otoplasty:

Some people have ears that stand out from their head further than normal. This is usually congenital, and anatomically is due to either an unfurled **antihelical** fold, a deep **conchal bowl,** or both. Many children are viciously teased by their peers because of their prominent ears. Surgical correction of the ears is a relatively simple and very satisfying operation. Interestingly, many 3rd-party payers feel this is "cosmetic" surgery and refuse to pay for it. They seem to ignore the tremendous difference between the person who looks normal and wants to look better (cosmetic surgery) and the person who looks abnormal and wants to look normal (reconstructive surgery). No child should be denied this operation if it is desired and the ears fall outside normal measurements. Hopefully, 3rd-party payers can be made to understand the difference in this case between "cosmetic" and "reconstructive" surgery.

73

Questions, Section #12

1. The most important part of any rhinoplasty is maintaining or improving the _____.

2. The first principle in the management of soft tissue wounds is _____.

Answers

1. AIRWAY
2. METICULOUS REAPPROXIMATION

If you die tomorrow, your residents would remember that you were a great guy for about six months. On the next Monday, your patients would be in someone else's office demanding service, angry that they were not getting it. And the only people who would miss you would be your family.

Josef E. Fischer, MD

A discussion of salivary glands should consider both **the major (parotid, submandibular, and sublingual) glands** as well as the minor salivary glands. It is estimated that normal individuals have **750-1000 minor salivary glands located submucosally** from the lips to the trachea.

First, consider bilateral salivary gland enlargement. Viral infection, mumps, and human immunodeficiency virus (HIV) are the most common causes. In addition, patients with autoimmune disorders may have salivary dysfunction (dry mouth), dry eyes, and arthritis. (A cluster syndrome known as Sjögren's disease is frequently associated with parotid enlargement.) Diagnosis is based not only on history and physical, but also on **serologic studies (SSA and SSB)**.

Bacterial parotitis is almost always caused by *Staphylococcus aureus* and presents with all the classic signs and symptoms of infection, which include **tumor (swelling), dolor (pain), calor (heat), and rubor (redness)**. Often, pus can be expressed from **Stensen's duct**. A potential cause is a salivary stone, although frequently the etiology is dehydration. Patients with bacterial parotitis generally do well when treated with hydration and high-dose intravenous antibiotics. Local applications of heat and **sialagogues** such as lemon drops are ancillary measures. Occasionally, they will need to be drained surgically.

Salivary gland stones (sialolithiasis) most commonly occur in the submandibular duct. They are usually, although not always, **radio-opaque.** They can occasionally be palpated, usually at the orifice of the duct adjacent to the **lingual frenulum**. When present, they can cause obstruction leading to **stasis with possible secondary bacterial infection.** Treatment is removal of the stone. The duct must be incised because the stone can't be milked out distally. Some institutions are investigating treatment with lithotripsy.

Masses often present in the salivary glands and need to be evaluated by an otolaryngologist. We often perform fine needle aspiration to determine whether a malignancy is present. In general, any lump in front or below the ear must be considered a parotid mass until proven otherwise. The parotid gland has a large amount of lymphoid

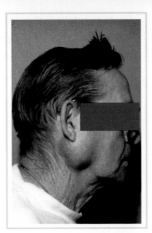

Figure 13.1.
Right parotid mass. Eighty-five percent of parotid neoplasms are benign, pleomorphic adenomas. However, 15% are malignant. Excisional biopsy requires superficial parotidectomy and facial nerve dissection. Open incisional biopsy is to be avoided except in unusual circumstances.

tissue, to which the lymphatics on the side of the head drain. The most common metastatic lesion to the parotid gland is squamous cell carcinoma, generally a metastasis from a cancer of the skin on the side of the head. Malignant melanoma on the ear or scalp also metastasizes to the lymph nodes in the parotid. There are a variety of diagnostic studies that can be performed. Physical exam, radiographic imaging, and fine needle aspiration are adequate for diagnosing 95% of parotid masses. However, surgical removal with superficial parotidectomy remains the final diagnostic step of choice. Parotid masses are usually resected with a superficial parotidectomy for 2 reasons: First, it is quite easy to damage the facial nerve unless it is traced out from its origin throughout its entire course in the gland. Second, the most common kinds of salivary tumors tend to recur, and this procedure allows the surgeon to get a good margin of tissue around the tumor and achieve a decreased recurrence rate. It is important that masses in this region not be **enucleated** because injudicious excision can result in both facial nerve injury and recurrent tumor.

A Few Basic Principles about Salivary Gland Tumors:

The larger the salivary gland, the less likely the tumor is to be malignant. Thus, a mass in the parotid has only a 15% chance of being a malignant tumor, but a mass in the sublingual gland has a 75% chance of being a malignant tumor. Masses in the submandibular gland have about a 50/50 chance of being malignant. The most common benign tumor of the salivary glands is a **pleomorphic adenoma (mixed tumor)**. The most common malignant tumors are **adenoid cystic carcinoma** and **mucoepidermoid carcinoma**. Adenoid cystic carcinoma has a strong propensity to invade nerves and track along them. This is obviously significant because the 7th nerve tracks right through the parotid gland. The lingual and hypoglossal nerves are very near the submandibular gland.

Questions, Section #13

1. The 4 classic signs and symptoms of an infection are

   _____,_____,_____,

   and_____.

2. Bacterial parotitis is most commonly caused by _____.

3. A lump in front of or below the ear is to be considered a _____ until proven otherwise.

4. The most common tumor in the parotid gland is benign and is a _____.

5. The treatment of tumors of the parotid gland includes _____ with complete dissection of the facial nerve.

Answers

1. PAIN (DOLOR), SWELLING (TUMOR), REDNESS (RUBOR), HEAT (CALOR)
2. S. AUREUS
3. PAROTID MASS
4. PLEOMORPHIC ADENOMA
5. SUPERFICIAL PAROTIDECTOMY

Thyroid cancer can be a confusing subject. **Thyroid nodules** are so common as to preclude removal in each patient who presents with them. Otolaryngologists therefore try to select nodules for removal that have a higher chance of being cancerous. A fine needle aspirate (FNA) that shows malignant cells is obviously an indication for sur-

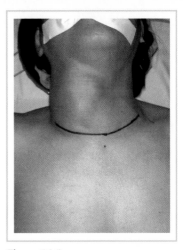

Figure 14.1.

Notice the large neck mass. In this case, it is from a benign thyroid goiter.

gery, as is any evidence of metastasis. If the lab report on the needle aspirate comes back benign and the patient doesn't have any other risk factors, you can be pretty certain of a benign diagnosis. If the lab report is inconclusive, however, you must press on. An ultrasound test will tell you if there are multiple nodules present. If multiple nodules are found, some otolaryngologists classify this as a **multinodular goiter** and do not operate. If you find a single (on ultrasound), inconclusive (on FNA) nodule, you may elect to try to suppress the nodule with oral **thyroid supplementation**. If any risk factors (see below) are present, you may consider operating on the nodule to get a definitive diagnosis. **Thyroid scans** have become less useful in the diagnostic workup of nodules with the development and refinement of fine needle aspiration.

Many more women than men have thyroid nodules, but a nodule in a male has a higher risk of being cancerous than a nodule in a female. Older people also develop more nodules than younger people. A nodule in a person younger than 40 years old has a higher chance of being cancer than a nodule in a person over 40. People who received radiation as children are also at increased risk of developing thyroid cancer.

The **4 major types of thyroid cancer** are **papillary, follicular** (including the **Hürthle cell** variant), **medullary,** and **anaplastic,** listed in increasing order of aggressiveness and decreasing order of frequency.

Papillary Carcinoma:

Approximately 80% of thyroid cancers are papillary. These may have a **follicular component,** but any amount of papillary component means the tumor will behave like a papillary tumor. These tumors **often metastasize** to neck lymph nodes, and **can be multifocal** in the gland. Lymph node masses don't appear to affect survival. Histologically, they have **clear nuclei** (Orphan Annie **cells**), and may have **psammoma** bodies. Factors predictive of a better prognosis include size smaller than 1.5 cm and absence of thyroid gland capsule involvement. For unknown reasons, this disease follows a much more indolent course when discovered in people under age 30-40 than when found in people older than 40. Thus, patients under 30 ultimately live longer. This may be one of the reasons why patients younger than 30 also have a higher recurrence rate.

80 Treatment

In the past, **lobectomy** and **isthmectomy** have been used. Newer evidence from a study by Mazzaferri and colleagues suggests that **total thyroidectomy,** when compared to subtotal, may significantly decrease the local recurrence rate (18% versus 7%) and ultimately the number of deaths (from 1.5% to 0.03%). This study also pointed out that treatment of patients with **radioactive iodine** and **thyroid hormone suppression** decreased the incidence of recurrence from 11% to 3% compared with those treated with thyroid suppression alone. There was, however, no difference in the number of deaths between these 2 groups. If neck masses are present, a **modified neck dissection** is indicated. Interestingly, no significant difference in recurrence has been shown between neck dissection and node plucking. The lower incidence of recurrence and death in total thyroidectomy must be weighed against the risk of **hypoparathyroidism** and **recurrent laryngeal nerve paralysis.** This risk obviously varies with each surgeon.

Follicular Carcinoma:

Approximately 15% of thyroid cancer is follicular. Two major types are **microinvasive** and **macroinvasive.** The surgical specimen of all thyroid cancers must be sectioned completely to determine if the tumor capsule or any blood vessels are invaded. This invasion is **pathognomonic,** and can't be determined by a fine needle aspirate. The cells may also look fairly benign on fine needle aspirate, so many specimens come back as "consistent with adenoma, cannot rule out follicular carcinoma." This tumor metastasizes via the blood. A variant of it is called Hürthle cell carcinoma.

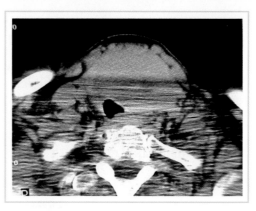

Figure 14.2.

This radiograph demonstrates invasion of the trachea with airway compression by a thyroid neoplasm.

Treatment

Follicular carcinoma has a higher affinity for radioactive iodine than does papillary carcinoma. Since iodine is concentrated in normal thyroid tissue, an attempt to remove all thyroid tissue allows a higher dose to be given to the mass. Total thyroidectomy (or at a very minimum, almost total) is therefore considered the treatment of choice. Postoperative radioactive iodine and thyroid suppression are then given.

81

Medullary Carcinoma:

Medullary carcinoma accounts for 6-10% of all thyroid cancer. There are **2 forms: familial (10-20%) and sporadic.** The tumor tends to be bilateral. The **parafollicular or C-cells** are the cell of origin. The familial form is a component of multiple endocrine neoplasms (MEN) IIa and IIb. MEN IIa is **parathyroid adenoma**, medullary carcinoma, and **pheochromocytoma.** MEN IIb doesn't have the parathyroid component and also has a **Marfanoid habitus** and mucosal neuromas. All patients with medullary carcinoma should get a urinary **metanephrine screen.** If this is positive, the pheochromocytoma should be found and excised first. All **1st-degree relatives** of patients with medullary carcinoma should be tested for **calcitonin level. Currently it has been demonstrated that**

the RET proto-oncogene is positive in most patients with this disease. This oncogene can be detected by a blood test.

Total thyroidectomy is indicated if they have abnormal studies. Interestingly, the calcitonin level doesn't always go down after total thyroidectomy. If it does, the patient can be followed up with pentagastrin infusion studies. Medullary carcinoma metastasizes to the cervical lymph nodes 50-60% of the time. It may also characteristically produce **amyloid** that stains green with congo red.

Treatment

Most authors recommend subtotal or total thyroidectomy with elective neck dissections. In patients with a neck mass, a modified neck dissection that encompasses all the involved levels of disease should be removed. In patients with the familial form, only abnormal parathyroid glands should be removed. A total thyroidectomy is always indicated in these familial patients. C-cells don't take up radioactive iodine, thus this modality of ancilliary treatment can not be used.

Anaplastic Carcinoma:

This is a rare tumor with a terrible prognosis. The surgeon's role is often limited to biopsy and securing the airway. These tumors are rarely resectable, and are often treated with radiotherapy for want of anything better.

Lymphoma:

Thyroid lymphoma can be difficult to differentiate from anaplastic carcinoma because of its rapid growth, which often produces airway compromise. Lymphomas typically arise in patients with a background of Hashimoto's thyroiditis, an autoimmune condition characterized by lymphocytic infiltration. Rapid diagnosis and institution of appropriate therapy is necessary to prevent airway obstruction.

This brief discussion on thyroid cancer should be distinguished from a discourse on surgery of the thyroid gland, which would include, for example, such subjects as surgery for hyperthyroidism (such as can occur with a toxic nodular goiter and Graves' disease). These conditions can also be treated medically, but further discussion here is beyond the scope of this book.

Questions, Section #14

1. The most common type of thyroid cancer is _____.

2. The 2nd most common type of thyroid cancer is _____.

3. The treatment of follicular cancer involves surgery plus
    _____.

4. Patients with medullary carcinoma should have a urinary
    _____ screen.

5. The thyroid tumor with the worst prognosis is _____
    carcinoma.

6. The first step in the diagnostic evaluation of a thyroid nodule after
    the history and physical is usually _____.

7. Medullary carcinoma of the thyroid can produce amyloid. When
    stained with congo red and looked at through a polarizing micro-
    scope, this appears _____.

Answers
1. PAPILLARY
2. FOLLICULAR
3. RADIOACTIVE IODINE
4. METANEPHRINE
5. ANAPLASTIC
6. NEEDLE ASPIRATION
7. GREEN

Head and Neck Cancer in Primary Care:

Diagnosis and management of head and neck cancer is a large topic. In this chapter we hope to provide you some background information and a few case studies to help. There are some things you must remember in the primary care setting, where you're most likely to be. First of all, an adult patient with a lump in the neck and no easily explainable reason for it should be considered to have cancer until that can be ruled out. Obviously,

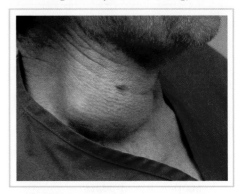

Figure 15.1.

This patient has a squamous cell carcinoma of the hypotharynx but presented to the primary care physician with a large upper neck mass. Fine Needle aspiration confirmed it to be squamous cell carcinoma.

this doesn't mean a child with strep throat and bilateral neck adenopathy, but it certainly does include a 60-year-old smoker who notices a lump while shaving. In the past, a physician would often biopsy a lump in a patient's neck and find that the lump was squamous cell carcinoma. The doctor would then take the patient back to the operating room for endoscopy and find that the patient actually had a **pyriform sinus squamous cell carcinoma** that had already metastasized to the neck. The problem with this scenario is that the patient's chance of survival may have been decreased because the neck was biopsied before definitive treatment of the primary, which, in this case, would have been resection of the tumor and a neck dissection followed by radiation therapy. This patient would need a complete head and neck exam, followed by triple endoscopy, before biopsy of the neck mass. If a needle aspirate is performed on a lump in the neck, it won't decrease the patient's chance of survival. The discovery of a squamous cell carcinoma on fine needle aspiration would tell you that you must look harder to find the primary.

Other patients who should be referred for laryngeal examination are those who have been hoarse for more than 2 weeks. The most common cause of hoarseness is an upper respiratory infection (URI) with edema (swelling) of the true vocal cords. This often lasts several weeks, but it rarely lasts 6 weeks. Six weeks of hoarseness in an adult is considered to be cancer of the larynx until proven otherwise. Other causes of hoarseness include inflammation from **gastroesophageal reflux disorder (GERD)**, allergic rhinitis causing postnasal drip, **laryngeal papillomatosis**, vocal cord nodules, vocal cord polyps, and **unilateral vocal cord paralysis**. However, patients who have become hoarse for no apparent reason should be referred without the 2-week waiting time.

Remember that allergic rhinitis causing postnasal drip and vocal cord inflammation is usually treated with intranasal steroid sprays. GERD, which can also give a feeling of having something stuck in the throat, is treated with antireflux measures. These include not eating within 3-4 hours of going to sleep, avoiding caffeine and alcohol (especially at night), and avoiding aspirin or nonsteroidal anti-inflammatory medications (including over-the-counter ones). You can also recommend that these patients elevate the head of their bed on bricks (extra pillows don't count) and take an antacid before bedtime. If they still have symptoms, they are usually started on an H2 blocker such as ranitidine or cimetidine. Proton pump inhibitors may be used in recalcitrant cases. Remember: Laryngeal examination is required before making these diagnoses and prescriptions.

85

A patient who may have cancer might also present to a primary care physician with pain in the throat or pain in the ear (**otalgia**) that has no obvious cause. The pharynx and hypopharynx are innervated by the 9th and 10th nerves. These also send branches to the ear, and sometimes a cancer in the throat can send referred pain to the ear. If a patient comes in with ear pain and the ear looks normal to you, it probably is normal and the pain is probably being caused by some other otolaryngologic problem. The most common cause of ear pain with a normal ear exam **is temporomandibular joint (TMJ) syndrome**. This is an inflammation of the joint of the jaw and can be diagnosed by pain on palpation of the joint (just in front of the **tragus**) when the patient opens and closes the jaw. If the joint is not tender and there is no other obvious cause of ear pain, the patient needs further evaluation. Likewise, difficulty in swallowing (**dysphagia**), pain on swallowing (**odynophagia**), or a **persistent oral ulcer** may be due to cancer. Patients with these symptoms should see an otolaryngologist. Sometimes a cancer in the nasopharynx can obstruct one of the Eustachian tubes, causing a **unilateral serous otitis (fluid in middle ear) in an adult**. The most common cause of this condition is simply a URI, but a unilateral serous otitis without a clear history of a cold must be referred for nasopharyngoscopy.

Occasionally, patients will present with a superficial lymph node located in the posterior triangle of the neck (behind the **sternocleidomastoid muscle**). Most commonly, this is a swollen lymph node secondary to some type of skin infection or inflammation on the scalp, so you should check the scalp carefully in such a case. Sometimes, however, this can be something as serious as a lymphoma. Usually, upper aerodigestive tract squamous cell carcinoma doesn't initially spread to the posterior triangle nodes, but, in rare cases, this can occur—especially with nasopharyngeal cancer. Physicians can be tempted to remove this superficial node of the neck in the office. However, these superficial posterior neck nodes should not be surgically addressed, except by someone very familiar with head and neck surgery: The **spinal accessory nerve** runs over the top of these nodes and can very easily be damaged if the doctor is not experienced in doing this kind of surgery.

You can also be easily fooled by discovering a lump in front of or below the ear. This most commonly represents a parotid neoplasia, the most common of which is the benign mixed tumor (pleomorphic adenoma). A mass in this area, however, can be something as superficial as an **epidermal inclusion cyst**, or something more serious—such as lymphoma. The problem with this particular area is that it is quite difficult to distinguish between something that is merely subcutaneous versus something that is in the parotid gland. The **ascending ramus of the mandible** is immediately deep to the parotid gland, thus a mass may be well within the substance of the gland; however, it can feel very superficial because there is a solid background immediately behind it. Well-intentioned surgeons, thinking this was a sebaceous cyst, have ventured into removing one of these lumps and found they unexpectedly need to go deep to the parotid fascia. If you ever find yourself in this position,

Surgery is a lot like sailing...the more exciting it is, the worse you are at doing it.

H. C. Pillsbury III, MD

you should immediately back out. This isn't the time for surgical hero-ics—remember the facial nerve! In situations such as this, it is better to refer the patient to an otolaryngologist.

Review

Like your 6th-grade teacher used to say, "Let's review." Since most doctors are in some type of primary care specialty, it is important to know when to refer a patient to a specialist in diseases of the head and neck for any symptoms that suggest the **possibility of cancer:**

- **a mass in the neck**

- **hoarseness for 2 weeks or more**

- **pain in the ear (otalgia), pain in the throat on swallowing (odynophagia), or difficulty swallowing (dysphagia)**

- **a lump below or in front of the ear**

- **a persistent oral ulcer**

- **unilateral serous otitis**

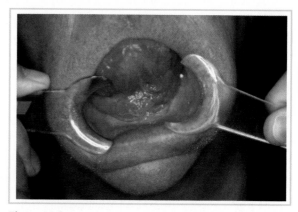

Almost all (95%) head and neck cancer is squamous cell carcinoma. The cancer originates from the **cuboidal cells** along the basement membrane of the mucosa. Under the microscope, the cancerous cells appear flat, so the cancer is called squamous (from the Latin *squama*, "a scale or plate-like structure") cell carcinoma. It occurs most

Figure 15.2.

Carcinoma of the floor of the mouth. Mucosal tumors of the upper aerodigestive tract are almost always squamous cell cancer and occur as a result of exposure to tobacco and alcohol. Unfortunately, tumors are often discovered late, making cure problematic.

often in middle-aged to elderly people who have exposed their upper aerodigestive tract mucosa to the carcinogens in cigarette smoke and ethanol. These carcinogenic agents act in a synergistic manner—that is, each promotes the occurrence of the cancer, but the combined effect is greater than the sum of the two. It follows that if a person gets one cancer, he or she may get another one in a different part of the upper aerodigestive tract (esophagus and lungs). Indeed, additional cancers are found in 10-20% of the patients who present with head and neck cancer.

Endoscopy Diagnosis and Treatment:

A full ENT exam is performed. In addition, fiberoptic or formal endoscopy in the operating room is performed.

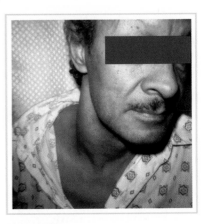

One reason for this is to evaluate the size and extent of the primary tumor (the original mucosal tumor, the source of the metastases likely to be found in the neck). Many patients present with a mass in the neck, and you will use endoscopy to locate the primary tumor. Sometimes the primary is very small, while the neck metastasis is very large. About 10% of the time in this situation, the primary tumor can't be found—this is called "**the unknown primary**."

Figure 15.3.

Mass occurring in mid-portion of right neck in a man with a past history of tobacco usage. This most likely represents metastatic squamous cell cancer from a primary site somewhere in the head and neck. Diagnostic workup includes head and neck examination, CT scan imaging, and fine needle aspiration biopsy.

A 2nd reason to perform endoscopy is to look for **second primaries**.

The 3rd reason to use endoscopy is to take a small piece of tissue with biopsy forceps to obtain a tissue diagnosis of cancer. Otolaryngologists use **rigid endoscopes** more than other specialists do because they make it easier to get a good biopsy specimen. (Rigid scopes are also the scope of choice for treatment of foreign body aspiration.)

Rigid endoscopy is usually done under general anesthesia for better relaxation and patient comfort. If the tumor is in the oral cavity, base of the tongue, or oral pharynx, it is palpated as well. The procedure usually takes less than an hour, and the patient may go home the same day. Overnight observation may be necessary if the patient has a large cancer of the larynx and there is a risk that the swelling caused by the procedure may obstruct the already compromised airway.

Diagnosis and Treatment:

Once the patient has been "scoped," what do you do next? Remember that endoscopy is used to evaluate the size of the tumor, including estimation of the 3rd dimension (depth). In general, T1 cancers measure less than 2 cm, T2 cancers are 2-4 cms, T3 are larger than 4 cm, and T4 are massive. Cancer of the larynx is usually smaller at presentation, and a different staging system is used. Little tumors without metastases do well and large or metastatic tumors do poorly. Unfortunately, though, 60-75% of patients don't present until the tumor is large or metastatic.

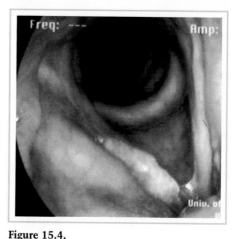

Figure 15.4.

Early squamous cell cancer of the vocal cord arising in a smoker. This patient presented with voice change and hoarseness. Early detection and appropriate treatment will cure essentially all of these individuals.

In general, T1 and T2 cancers respond well to surgery or radiation therapy with good results (75-80% 5-year survival). For larger or metastatic lesions, combined surgery and radiation therapy is usually recommended and the prognosis is poorer (15-35% 5-year survival). In addition, chemotherapy seems to synergize with irradiation and has become an important adjunct in the treatment of head and neck cancer.

When head and neck cancer patients receive radiation therapy as part of their treatment, it is usually given once per day for 6 weeks, although some physicians use twice-per-day protocols. It is generally felt that 5600 rads (centigray [cGy]) is a minimum dose for a neck with microscopic disease. If there is a big, bulky tumor somewhere, the dose may go up to 7000 cGy. Implants (**brachytherapy**) may be placed to deliver a very high, localized dose. Radiation therapy also dries the major and minor salivary glands. Since teeth remineralize with the minerals in saliva, they are very prone to decay during and after this therapy. If a patient has teeth in very poor condition, all the teeth are extracted before the patient begins radiation therapy. This is called a total odontectomy, and has nothing at all to do with removing the odontoid process.

Metastasis:

Squamous cell carcinoma tends to metastasize early to the lymph nodes of the neck before going to the lung, liver, bone, and brain. A chest x-ray is obtained to be certain the patient has neither metastasis nor a second tumor (which is more likely) in the lung. If the tumor has metastasized to the lungs or liver, the role of surgery is limited to palliation. If the metastases are confined to the lymph nodes of the neck (the most common scenario), then a neck dissection—removing lymph nodes from the neck—is performed at the time of surgery. The lymph nodes are nestled in fat and wrapped in fascia. **Selective neck dissection (SND)** involves removing only nodes, fat, and fascia most likely involved by metastasis. A **radical neck dissection (RND)** is performed when bulky metastasis demands radical surgery and includes **removal of the sternomastoid muscle, internal jugular vein, and spinal accessory nerve**. The main deformity that results from most head and neck surgery is caused by the surgery done to remove the primary, so the term "radical" should be used to describe only the neck dissection, not the entire cancer-removing procedure.

The intern suffers not only from inexperience, but also from over experience. He has in his short term of service, responsibilities which are too great for him. He becomes accustomed to act without preparation and he acquires a confidence in himself and a self complacency which may be useful in time of emergency, but which tend to blind him to his inadequacy and warp his career.

W. H. Halstead

Questions, Section #15

1. By far, the most common cancer of the upper aerodigestive tract is _____.

2. Cigarette smoke and ethanol work in a _____ manner to promote cancer.

3. People who have one cancer of the upper aerodigestive tract may often have another, which is one of the reasons why _____ is performed.

4. Evaluation of the actual size of a tumor, as well as taking a biopsy, are two other reasons why_____ is performed before final treatment of a head and neck cancer.

5. Small head and neck cancers can often be treated with either _____ or _____.

6. Large head and neck cancers are often treated with _____ and _____.

7. Squamous cell carcinoma of the head and neck usually metastasizes to the lymph nodes in the _____ before going to other sites.

8. One key to happiness in the 3rd year of medical school is to _____.

9. A radical neck dissection (RND) involves removing the sternocleidomastoid muscle, the spinal accessory nerve, and the_____, which are intimately related to the lymphatic structures of the neck.

10. Total odontectomy involves _____.

11. Radiation therapy dries up the _____ glands.

12. A mass in the neck may be a _____ from a cancer somewhere in the upper aerodigestive tract.

13. A patient who is hoarse for more than 2 weeks may have _____ of the larynx.

14. A patient with a lump below or in front of the ear may have a tumor of the _____ gland and need to see an otolaryngologist.

15. A persistent oral ulcer may be the first sign of a _____.

16. When there is a normal ear exam, pain in the ear may be caused by a _____ in the pharynx.

17. Persistent unilateral serous otitis media may be caused by a _____ in the nasopharynx obstructing the Eustachian tube.

18. Parotid masses feel superficial, because the parotid gland is immediately superficial to the_____ of the mandible.

Answers

1. SQUAMOUS CELL CARCINOMA
2. SYNERGISTIC
3. TRIPLE ENDOSCOPY
4. ENDOSCOPY
5. SURGERY, RADIATION THERAPY
6. SURGERY, RADIATION THERAPY
7. NECK
8. READ FOR AN HOUR EVERY DAY
9. JUGULAR VEIN
10. REMOVING ALL THE TEETH
11. SALIVARY
12. METASTASIS
13. CANCER
14. PAROTID
15. CANCER
16. CANCER
17. CANCER
18. ASCENDING RAMUS

The great majority of skin cancers arising on the skin of the face, scalp, and neck are **basal cell carcinoma**, followed by squamous cell carcinoma, then **malignant melanoma**. Basal cell carcinoma is very common and most often occurs on the face, so the otolaryngologist-facial plastic surgeon sees many cases.

The typical basal cell carcinoma is a **nodular lesion with a raised, pearly-white border**. These are usually brought to the doctor's attention before they become very large. They don't metastasize and can be treated in a variety of ways. Dermatologists may freeze or curette them. Facial plastic surgeons tend to excise them with a small margin and do a meticulous closure of the defect. Occasionally, the defect will require the rotation of a small local flap.

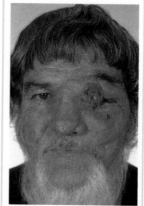

Figure 16.1.

Very large basal cell carcinoma of the facial skin. Note the rolled edges with central ulceration, indicating subepithelial extension. Excision must ensure that the tumor is completely excised or recurrence is inevitable.

Another way of addressing these cancers involves **Mohs' fresh tissue chemosurgery technique**, in which the tumor is removed in layers and completely examined under a microscope to ensure complete removal. This takes significantly longer than any of the other methods, but the recurrence rate is lower when Mohs' technique is used. For this reason, certain tumors with a higher than usual chance of recurrence with conventional excisions may be better managed with Mohs' surgery. A basal cell carcinoma that **recurs** after primary treatment with either excision, electrodesiccation, curettage, or freezing is at higher risk for recurring after the 2nd course of treatment, so these patients will often undergo Mohs' surgery. Basal cell carcinomas that occur **near vital**

structures such as the eyelids, nose, or ears are also often treated with Mohs' surgery in order to preserve as much normal tissue as possible. **Morpheaform basal cell carcinoma** is a kind of basal cell carcinoma that has very indistinct borders, more like a yellow plaque than a raised nodular lesion. It is very difficult to excise without the use of histology, so this type of basal cell carcinoma is best suited to Mohs' surgery. In addition, a basal cell carcinoma that is **very large** on initial presentation also has a higher incidence of recurrence and should be considered for Mohs' surgery. Unfortunately, Mohs' surgery is costly, so the merits of each case must be considered individually.

Squamous cell carcinoma is more aggressive and generally requires excision of a larger margin than basal cell carcinoma to assume complete removal. This tumor can metastasize, although usually not early in its course. Evaluation of the neck nodes and careful follow up to detect early recurrence or metastasis is necessary. Larger tumors are usually treated with wide excision and neck dissection to remove any possible metastases.

Malignant Melanoma:

Malignant melanoma is a capricious tumor that affects patients of all ages and has a high mortality rate. There is mounting evidence that sun exposure in childhood is a strong risk factor. It is very common in Australia, and public education in that country has led to the widespread frequent wearing of broad-brimmed hats and use of sunscreen lotions among 50% of adults and children. If you're caucasian and have young children, be sure they're protected from the sun when outside in the summer and in warmer climates. Melanoma presents as a **pigmented lesion (mole)** that changes by either growth, changes in color or margin, ulceration, or bleeding, or is deeply pigmented or raised.

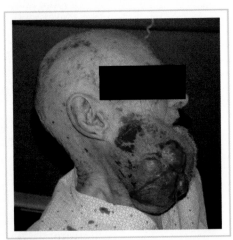

Figure 16.2.

This large neglected squamous cell carcinoma of the face is present in this homeless individual.

Melanoma begins in the epidermis and then invades the dermis. The depth of invasion is strongly predictive of spread and, ultimately, patient survival. The classification system includes thin (less than 0.76 mm invasion), thick (greater than 4.0 mm), and intermediate (greater than 0.76 mm and less than 4.0 mm). The risk of metastatic disease is less than 10% with thin but greater than 90% with thick. It's important that every physician keep a close lookout for darkly pigmented moles and those that have changed, that bleed, are raised, or have irregular margins. Early detection and excision are lifesaving.

Questions, Section #16

1. The most common types of skin cancer are _____, _____, and _____.

2. Most basal cell carcinomas are nodular in appearance, with very distinct borders, and are easily treatable. There is, however, a certain type that has very indistinct borders. This is called a

_____.

3. Certain basal cell carcinomas have a higher incidence of recurrence than others. These include _____, _____, and _____.

4. Some basal cell carcinomas may be very close to vital structures, such as the lower eyelid or the ala of the nose. In this case, maximum preservation of tissue is a consideration and these patients are candidates for _____ surgery.

5. Squamous cell carcinoma of the face is aggressive and can metastasize to the _____.

6. The metastatic potential of malignant melanoma depends on _____.

7. Signs of malignant melanoma are a mole that _____, _____, _____, and _____.

Answers

1. BASAL CELL, SQUAMOUS CELL, MALIGNANT MELANOMA
2. MORPHEAFORM CARCINOMA
3. RECURRENT, LARGE (GREATER THAN 2 CM), AND MORPHEAFORM
4. MOHS'
5. CERVICAL LYMPH NODES
6. TUMOR THICKNESS
7. IS DARKLY PIGMENTED, RAISED, BLEEDING, CHANGING, HAS IRREGULAR MARGINS

A high percentage of illnesses affecting children involve the ears, nose, and throat. Nearly all oto-laryngologists treat children in their practices, and some treat only children. This chapter will be useful to you in your pediatric rotation as well as any ENT exposure you might have. An excellent library reference on pediatric otolaryngology is the two-volume text by Bluestone and Stool. You should refer to it often during your pediatric rotation.

The most common pediatric disorder seen by the otolaryngologist and pediatrician is **otitis media**, so it's important to understand the spectrum of this disease. This is presented in this book in chapter 5, "Otitis Media."

Tonsillectomy:

In the past, the indication for (reason to perform) a **tonsillectomy** was the presence of tonsils. In the pre-antibiotic era, it was the only treatment available. Now, otolaryngologists have refined patient selection and, for the most part, we do tonsillectomies on patients with recurrent or chronic tonsillitis, obstructive sleep apnea, asymmetric tonsils, and peritonsillar abscess.

Recurrent Tonsillitis:

Some children have several bouts of tonsillitis per year that require evaluation by a physician. In treating **recurrent tonsillitis**, you should obtain culture documentation of *Group A, ß hemolytic strep*, if possible. Published AAO-HNS *2000 Clinical Indicators Compendium* suggest that tonsillectomy is indicated if children present with 3 or more infections per year despite adequate medical therapy. Some physicians feel that if a child misses 2 weeks of school in a year because of tonsillitis, the tonsils should come out. However, each patient is different, and the final decision should be an agreement between the patient or parents and doctor.

Chronic Tonsillitis:

Chronic low-grade infection of the tonsils can occur in older children, adolescents, and adults.

Interestingly, there is an increasing awareness that hyperactivity may be associated with sleep apnea. These patients often have large **crypts** or spaces within the tonsils that collect food and **debris** and are difficult to sterilize with antibiotics. The lymph nodes in the neck are usually inflamed from constant tonsillar infection. Sometimes, the

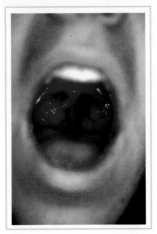

Figure 17.1.

Massive tonsil hypertrophy. Indications for tonsillectomy include recurrent episodes of tonsillitis or chronic upper airway obstruction resulting in sleep apnea. Enlargement without symptoms is not an indication for removal.

retained food and debris lead to chronic halitosis (bad breath). The typical history from these patients is that their sore throat gets better on antibiotics, but then comes back as soon as they stop taking their medication.

Obstructive Sleep Disorders:

Some patients may have e**nlarged tonsils** as well as an increased amount of soft tissue in their pharynx and hypopharynx. This leads to **chronic upper airway obstruction** due to enlarged tonsils and adenoids, and can result in **obstructive sleep apnea** in some children. **Daytime lethargy, obstructive symptoms, and nocturnal enuresis** are often associated with the condition. Interestingly, there is an increasing awareness that hyperactivity may be associated with sleep apnea. In severe—although rare—cases, cor pulmonale can result. Diagnosis is usually straightforward, based on history and physical, although a recorded sleep tape is frequently used as collaborative evidence. In some instances, a formal sleep study may be required. If the diagnosis of obstruction is correct, tonsillectomy and adenoidectomy (T and A) is often curative.

A particularly severe form of sleep apnea occurs in children with **Down syndrome**. Surgery on these children carries increased risk and requires specialized anesthetic care.

Asymmetric Tonsils:

Asymmetric tonsils are usually due to **recurrent scarring from infections**, but they may harbor tumors (such as lymphoma) and should be removed for **pathologic examination**. Remember that asymmetry of the tonsils also may be apparent—that is, not real—because of asymmetry of the soft palate and anterior pillars.

Peritonsillar Abscess:

An abscess that collects in the potential **space between the pharyngeal constrictor and the tonsil** itself is termed a **peritonsillar abscess** or "quinsy." These patients present with a history of having had a sore throat for a few days, which has now become significantly worse on one side. The classic signs of a peritonsillar abscess are **fullness of the anterior tonsillar pillar, deviated uvula**, "hot-potato voice," and severe **dysphagia**. Most of these patients also have **trismus (inability to open the jaw)** to some extent. Treatment is either aspiration with a large needle or incision and drainage done under local anesthesia. A 1-inch incision is made in the superior part of the anterior tonsillar pillar. A hemostat is used to open up the incision into the peritonsillar abscess, and the abscess is drained. Usually, the patient is given high-dose intravenous penicillin and sent home on oral antibiotics. Some patients will suffer only 1 episode in their lives, but if a patient has 2 or more episodes, a tonsillectomy is usually recommended. In a child, general anesthesia may be necessary to drain the abscess. If so, you should consider performing a tonsillectomy at the same time, especially if there is a history of recurrent or chronic infections or airway obstructions. Many surgeons routinely prefer urgent tonsillectomy because they feel this most effectively drains the abscess as well as prevents recurrence.

99

Adenoidectomy:

The **adenoids** are **lymphoid tissue** that hang off the posterior pharyngeal wall and roof of the nasopharynx, just behind the **soft palate** and bilaterally adjacent to the **torus tubarius**. When the adenoids are enlarged, nasal obstruction and chronic mouth-breathing ensue. **Adenoiditis** can be an underlying cause of otitis media as a result of secondary eustachian tube dysfunction and the proximity of a bacteria reservoir. In children, it can also be associated with chronic sinusitis. Adenoidectomy is often performed in children older than 2 years who have recurrent acute otitis media or otitis media with effusion, especially if effusion has returned after tube insertion. Tonsillectomy is also performed for children who snore loudly or have apnea with nasal obstruction. Adenoids usually atrophy with puberty, although they can be enlarged in teenagers and adults.

Foreign Bodies in the Ear and Nose:

Let's face it: Children seem to have a propensity for putting things into just about any orifice possible. Thus, they'll often place things such as pebbles, erasers, small toys, etc., into their external auditory canal. Treating this is usually a fairly benign process that can be dealt with in a non-emergent manner, but the exception to the rule is if there is a strong possibility of damage to the middle or inner ear. If this has occurred, the child may have lost sensorineural hearing, and may also be dizzy. Another exception is if the foreign body is alive! It is important to kill insects in the ear canal (usually by drowning in drops of olive oil is a good choice) before removal. These children should be referred immediately to an otolaryngologist. Most commonly, the foreign body remains in the lateral part of the external auditory canal. Remember that these young patients often become uncooperative and may require general anesthesia for the simple removal of the object, especially if prior attempts have been made to remove it. Therefore, unless certain, easy, nontraumatic, removal of the foreign body is completely assured, referral to an otolaryngologist is recommended.

Children also like to put foreign bodies in their nose. This invariably results in **unilateral, foul-smelling, purulent rhinorrhea**. Parents will often report that their child "smells bad." The key here is that the rhinorrhea is on only one side. (If it were due to a cold or a sinus infection, it should be bilateral.) Occasionally, removal will require general anesthesia, but topical anesthesia and vasoconstrictive nose drops may shrink the swelling sufficiently to

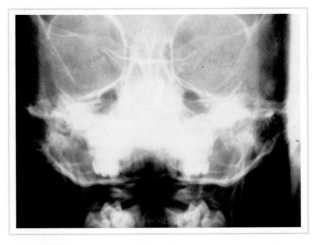

Figure 17.2.

Radiograph demonstrating a button battery in the nasal cavity of a child with profuse unilateral rhinorrhea. Button batteries can leak caustic fluid and result in serious burns.

aid in removal. You must be aware of the potential problems caused by button batteries. These objects can cause severe burns and should be removed emergently to prevent or minimize long-term complications. If lodged in the esophagus, they can cause fatal perforation with **mediastinitis**.

Stridor:

Children are also commonly referred to the otolaryngologist for **stridor**, high-pitched, noisy respiration that is a sign of respiratory obstruction. Stridor can be caused by a number of conditions, and among the most life-threatening conditions associated with it are **acute epiglottitis**, **croup**, or **foreign body aspiration**.

Acute Epiglottitis:

This is an infection of the supraglottic structures that causes such severe swelling of the epiglottis that it blocks the airway. It is fulminant and usually caused by *Haemophilus influenzae* type B organisms. This fatal disease was common 20 years ago, but the incidence has decreased dramatically with widespread use of the *H. influenzae* vaccine. The typical affected child is 3-6 years old and septic. Often, the child was breathing normally just hours earlier. You'll notice that the child is stridorous, as well as leaning forward and drooling because it hurts to swallow. If you suspect acute epiglottitis, call ENT, anesthesia, and pediatrics at once. Remember: If the child obstructs acutely, the airway can almost always be maintained with a bag and mask. Do not attempt to examine the child or force the child to lie back, because the agitation associated with the examination can precipitate sudden, complete obstruction. These cases are difficult and try the most skillful of anesthesiologists. Every effort must be made to expedite rapid transport to the operating room with as little manipulation as possible. If there is a reasonable amount of doubt as to the diagnosis, then an alternative is to have doctors from all 3 services accompany the patient to the radiology suite for a lateral soft tissue view of the neck. This is rarely done. Instead, doctors from all 3 services should accompany him or her to the operating room, where he or she can be masked down with an inhalation agent and intubated. An IV can then be started and blood cultures obtained.

Appropriate antibiotic therapy includes coverage for *H. influenzae* type B as well as for the much more rare *Staphylococcus aureus* organisms until final confirmation of the cause by blood cultures. Appropriate double-drug therapy would be ceftriaxone and oxacillin. Appropriate single-drug therapy would be cefuroxime, which can be continued by mouth later. The patient is usually extubated within 48-72 hours after confirmation of resolution by laryngoscopy.

Croup:

Croup should be **distinguished** from acute epiglottitis. Croup is the common name for **laryngotracheobronchitis**, a **viral infection of the upper airway** causing swelling in the subglottic area and stridor. It usually occurs in children 6 months - 3 years old who have had a prodromal URI usually for about a week. Patients are not

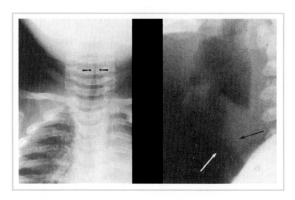

Figure 17.3.

This radiograph demonstrates steeplechase narrowing of the trachea in a young child with croup. See arrow.

septic but may have a low-grade fever. The stridor is high pitched and associated with a "barking" cough—often sounding like a seal. It doesn't hurt to swallow, so the patient isn't drooling; the epiglottis isn't swollen, so the patient isn't always leaning forward. The classic radiographic finding is the "steeple sign" showing subglottic narrowing on a chest or neck **x-ray**.

The treatment for croup is **humidity, oxygen, and if necessary, racemic epinephrine treatments, or steroids, or both**. Antibiotic therapy may be used if bacterial infection is suspected. If croup is severe, the child should be admitted to the hospital for observation. Intubation is rarely required. Rarely, children with subglottic stenosis will present with "recurrent croup". In these children evaluation by an otolaryngologist including direct laryngoscopy is required.

Foreign Bodies:

Foreign bodies can be another cause of stridor in children. Most commonly, it's caused by a foreign body that has been aspirated into the tracheobronchial tree—anything from coins to peanuts to Christmas tree light bulbs. (It's always important that small children aren't allowed access to such things as small toy parts, peanuts, raw carrot pieces, and other things of similar size.) Foreign bodies in the airway often prompt paroxysmal coughing and stridor that resolves, followed by wheezing, so it's critical that your diagnosis not be confused with asthma. Occasionally, there can be a symptom-free period after initial aspiration.

Small objects swallowed by children can also lodge in the hypopharynx or esophagus. Occasionally, the child will refuse to drink anything and may present with drooling. Sometimes, the patient will not eat, but will drink. In these cases, an x-ray is usually obtained and, under general anesthesia, a **rigid esophagoscope** is used to remove the foreign body from the esophagus. If the foreign body has been aspirated, then bronchoscopy is required. A problem with the aspiration of peanuts (which seems to be quite common) is that the oil and salt produce a chemical inflammation that causes the bronchial mucosa to swell, making removal difficult. Don't forget that a child may present with recurrent bouts of pneumonia, and this can be due to an aspirated foreign body that wasn't detected at the time of aspiration. Occasionally, bronchial ball valve obstruction will result in hyperinflation of one lung, which is visible on chest x-ray.

103

Subglottic Stenosis:

With the advent of modern neonatal intensive care, **subglottic stenosis** has become an increasingly common cause of stridor. It is most commonly caused by scarring from long-term placement of an endotracheal tube. Neonates seem to tolerate extended endotracheal intubation better than adults; however, after weeks and months of intubation, some of these patients may develop scarring in the subglottic area that causes a narrowing of the airway. This can occur acutely or over the course of several months. These patients present with stridor, which may be **biphasic** because it's due to a fixed obstruction in the larynx. (Children with subglottic stenosis are sometimes erroneously diagnosed as having asthma.)

If the subglottic stenosis is severe, there are several treatment options. The first option is to place a tracheostomy to bypass the obstruction. There are many problems associated with tracheostomy in infants, including delays in speech development, chronic mucous plugging, and even risk of death due to an obstructed tube. A better solution is to surgically enlarge the airway with a **cricoid split**. This can include simply making a cut in the cricoid ring and allowing it to expand while an endotracheal tube remains in the airway for a week to 10 days. If this is inadequate and the child still has some stenosis, or if the stenosis is so severe that a cricoid split might not be enough, a **laryngotracheal reconstruction** can be performed, in which pieces of rib cartilage are grafted into the front of the cricoid cartilage and upper tracheal rings and sometimes the back of the cricoid cartilage. These can be held in place with a stent for varying lengths of time. The chances of this working are good, especially if the stenosis wasn't extremely severe to begin with. Another way of treating mild stenosis involves using a laser to incise or excise the involved area. This has not met with good success, except in cases where the affected area was quite small and only minimal lasering was necessary.

Subglottic Hemangioma:

Another cause of stridor in children can be a **subglottic hemangioma**. Classically, 50% of these patients will have other associated head and neck hemangiomata, which will be visible on the skin. In some situations, these hemangiomas can be treated with a laser. Systemic steroids and interferon may play a role as well. Some pediatric otolaryngologists will do laser therapy without performing a tracheostomy, others prefer to have a tracheostomy. Obviously, this also depends on the size of the lesion

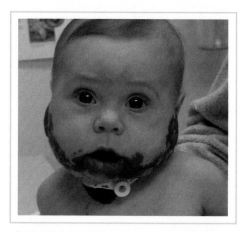

Figure 17.4.
This young child has a large hemangioma with cosmetic as well as functional symptoms.

and the size of the airway; occasional spontaneous involution can occur.

Vascular Rings:

Yet another cause of stridor in children is **vascular rings**, which may also be accompanied by periods of apnea. These cause compression of the trachea by either the innominate artery or any of the various persisting vascular rings that can occur embryologically. For example, a double-arched aorta may compress both the esophagus and the trachea. This diagnosis is generally made by visualizing an anterior compression of the trachea on bronchoscopy. A barium swallow will occasionally show an indentation behind the esophagus if there is a complete vascular ring present that encircles the esophagus and the trachea. The definitive diagnosis is made with either a CT scan or an MRI of the chest. If the symptoms are severe enough, treatment can include ligation of the offending vessel or rerouting. These conditions are fairly rare.

Laryngomalacia:

Perhaps the most common cause of persistent stridor in infants is **laryngomalacia**. Classically, this is associated with a floppy, omega-shaped epiglottis and is thought to be due to high-speed airflow through the narrow, redundant tissue of the supraglottic area. This is a diagnosis of exclusion, and more life-threatening causes of stridor must be ruled out first. If there are no apneic spells and the patient is otherwise asymptomatic, treatment is simply observation because these children will usually grow out of the condition. If the patient has apneic episodes or desaturates, then the supraglottic tissues can be trimmed or a tracheostomy can be performed. Other indications for surgical intervention include poor weight gain or failure to thrive. Interestingly, recent reports would indicate an association between GERD and laryngomalacia. This usually alleviates the stridor.

Neck Mass:

Another common reason for otolaryngologists to see children is the presence of a **neck mass**. Neck masses in children are most likely to be benign, compared with adults, in whom these masses are more likely to be malignant. They can be divided into **congenital, infectious, and neoplastic** categories.

Congenital Neck Masses:

One of the common congenital neck masses is a **cystic hygroma**, which is also known as a **lymphangioma** and occurs commonly in the neck region. It can be massive and extend up into the floor of the mouth or into the airway. These patients can need immediate intubation or a surgical airway at birth, if the neck mass is large enough to cause obstruction. Otherwise, the hygroma can usually be removed by elective surgery.

105

Another common cause of a neck mass in children is a **branchial cleft cyst**. These are found along the anterior border of the sternocleidomastoid muscle. This can occasionally become infected and swell, only to respond to antibiotic therapy, shrink, and then return later. Often these children are slightly older when they present for excision. In addition, a **thyroglossal duct cyst** can cause neck masses in children. These occur in the midline, usually over the thyrohyoid membrane. They are attached to the hyoid bone and move

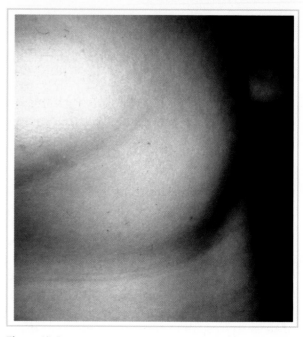

Figure 17.5.

Neck masses arising in children are usually benign (as opposed to adults, in whom they are usually malignant). This is a cystic hygroma, a congenital malformation of lymphatic vessels.

with swallowing. Treatment is by surgical excision with a **Sistrunk operation**, where the mid-portion of the hyoid bone is removed along with the cyst's stalk to the base of the tongue.

Infectious Neck Masses:

Infectious causes of neck masses in children are more common than congenital causes. Perhaps the most common reason for enlarged lymph nodes in a child is tonsillitis or pharyngitis. Occasionally, the lymph nodes themselves can become infected, usually with *Staphylococcus* or *Streptococcus* species (**cervical adenitis**). Patients are usually febrile, and the nodes are very tender to palpation. Occasionally, these lymph nodes may suppurate and require surgical drainage.

You should always consider cat-scratch disease when children present with **suppurative adenitis**. The patient's history of being scratched by a cat is the key to making this diagnosis. However, sometimes the child is unaware of the incident. These children are also afebrile, and the nodes are usually not tender, but there is redness and swelling.

Another condition that must always be considered in a child with swollen lymph nodes is **tuberculosis**. Classically, this occurs in multiple lymph nodes. The old word for tuberculosis lymph nodes in the neck was "scrofula." Workup includes a chest x-ray, a purified protein derivative (PPD) test, and a fine needle aspirate. In this case, the nodes are not treated with excision but, rather, with standard anti-tuberculosis medications.

Atypical tuberculosis is occasionally a cause of swollen lymph nodes in children. Generally, this is confined to 1 or 2 areas of the neck. The nodes are not usually painful, and the patient is not toxic. In atypical TB, the lymph nodes follow a somewhat predictable course wherein the skin overlying the lymph node becomes red and the lymph node appears to "stick to the skin." This may eventually lead to spontaneous drainage. However, excision of the lymph nodes is indicated if they do not respond to medical therapy.

Retropharyngeal cellulitis or abscess is an important infection in children. This is essentially a cervical adenitis that occurs in the space behind the pharynx. These patients may have an obvious amount of inflammation on the anterior spinal ligament, as well as up around the base of the skull, and can therefore present with a stiff neck (**meningismus**) and fever. It may be difficult to discriminate between this disease and meningitis. A lateral neck x-ray will usually show an increased thickness of the soft tissue just anterior to the spine. A CT scan is useful to image the exact location of the abscess or infected lymph node, which is then treated with intravenous antibiotics. Cellulitis will respond to antibiotics, but abscesses will require surgical incision and drainage, through either the mouth or neck. Sometimes, a patient's response to antibiotics will be so dramatic as to suggest that no true abscess was ever present, but simply a severe cervical adenitis that responded to appropriate therapy. Antibiotic coverage should include coverage for *S. aureus* organisms, anaerobes, and *H. influenzae* infection. Often there is such concern over the possibility of meningitis that a drug that penetrates the cerebrospinal fluid should be used. Adequate choices include cefuroxime or ticarcillin and clavulanate. Vancomycin should be considered if resistant organisms such as penicillin-resistant *Streptococcus pneumoniae* are suspected.

Malignant Neck Masses:

Malignant neck masses in children are rare, and include salivary gland malignancy, which is treated surgically. Tumors of the thyroid gland also occur, and may be accompanied by metastatic disease in the lymph nodes. **Lymphoma**, especially Hodgkin's, can present as cervical adenopathy.

Congenital Nasal Mass:

Very rarely, a child may be born with a congenital mass between the eyes and over the bridge of the nose **(nasion)**. This can be either a **dermoid cyst** or a **congenital herniation of the intracranial tissues (encephalocele** or **meningoencephalocele). Heterotopic brain tissue**, called glioma, is also possible and may not have a connection to the central nervous system (CNS). In making your diagnosis, you should obtain a CT scan to see if there is a **bony defect**. An MRI scan may also be quite helpful to determine whether there is simply a residual cord of tissue or whether there is a defect that allows either the meninges alone or the meninges and brain to protrude through the defect. These patients should be referred for surgical excision.

Tongue Tie:

Not uncommonly, children will have a very short lingual frenulum that prevents them from sticking out their tongue. This makes it especially hard to make certain sounds like "L" (and to eat an ice cream cone), but is easily corrected by incising the frenulum. It may present as difficulty in breast feeding in a neonate.

Rhinosinusitis:

All children (and adults) suffer from an occasional bout of rhinosinusitis. Most of these are viral and of short duration, and require no therapy. Parents, however, can be upset over the nasal drainage (often green, yellow, or gray), and especially upset that they can't leave their sick child in daycare because of the illness. It is important to reassure parents that these colds are normal, and to resist the temptation to treat mucus with antibiotics. Some children, however, will have persistent illness that lasts for weeks or months and is associated with fever. These patients may benefit from antibiotics directed toward common pathogens. Also, some children will benefit from adenoidectomy, and occasionally sinus aspiration or even surgery may be required.

Rarely, sinus infection can lead to orbital infection. If an abscess develops with visual change, **proptosis**, or loss of normal eye movement, urgent surgical drainage is required to prevent loss of vision. A diagnostic CT scan is required in suspected cases. These abscesses can often be drained successfully through an endoscopic approach, but an external incision (just medial to the medial canthus) may be required.

Questions, Section #17

1. Four indications for performing tonsillectomy are _____, _____, _____, and _____.

2. A 2-year-old child presents to your office with otitis media with effusion. The fluid has been present in his ears for 3 months despite treatment with a 3-week course of trimethoprim and sulfamethoxazole. His mother says that he's having trouble hearing. He has had 1 set of PE tubes in the past. You plan to place another set of PE tubes, and at this time you think that the child may benefit from an _____.

3. Unilateral, foul-smelling rhinorrhea in a child is most commonly due to a _____.

4. A 4-year-old child presents at the St. Elsewhere Emergency Room with inspiratory stridor and a fever of 103°F, and she is drooling and leaning forward. Her mother states that the child was well 4 hours ago, and she thinks that the child swallowed a stick because her throat hurts now and she was playing with small sticks in the yard outside. Your first concern is that this child may have _____.

5. You then call the anesthesiologist and pediatrician, but while waiting for them to arrive you notice that the child is starting to tire out. In fact, she becomes so tired from trying to breathe that she simply faints and ceases all attempts at respiration. The first thing you do for this child is _____.

6. Your next patient in the emergency room is a 1-year-old who presents with a chief complaint of stridor. He had a cold during this past week. On examination, he isn't sitting up and leaning forward and he isn't drooling. He does have inspiratory stridor, however. He does not have a fever, but he has a barking cough. The most likely diagnosis in this case is _____.

7. You therefore obtain soft tissue x-ray of the neck and a chest x-ray to look for the classic steeple sign. You are surprised when you find the child has actually aspirated a small metal object that appears to be the tip of a pen. Removal is with a rigid _____.

8. A multiloculated cystic neck mass in a newborn child that transilluminates is most probably a _____.

9. A midline neck mass in a child that moves when the child sticks out his tongue, but is otherwise not tender and is found in the area of the hyoid bone is most probably a _____.

10. A 2-year-old child presents to you with a high fever and large, painful, and inflamed left posterior triangle lymph nodes. The most likely diagnosis is _____.

11. Another 2-year-old child presents without fever and with no pain, but with large, firm lymph nodes in the posterior triangle of the neck. There are no lesions in the scalp seen on examination. In fact, the child seems to be almost oblivious to these nodes. The child does not have a cat, and hasn't been recently scratched by a cat or a dog. The most common cause of this type of neck mass in a child is _____.

12. A 2-year-old child presents to you with a fever of 103°F. His mother says he hasn't eaten anything all day and has vomited once. His neck is very stiff, and he won't move his head. He has had a cold over the last 3-4 days. You do an exam and find that his ears aren't infected and he won't open his mouth at all, and he still won't move his head. You obtain cerebrospinal fluid with a lumbar puncture (after noting the absence of papilledema on physical exam), and you send this to the lab. It returns with normal glucose and protein concentrations and no white blood cells. The opening and closing pressures are normal, and the fluid is quite clear. Every time you try to look in the patient's throat, he turns away, gags, and screams. You're thinking he may have cervical adenitis, so you order a _____.

13. The lateral neck x-ray shows increased soft tissue thickness in the prevertebral area, but the child's head is bent down, and it's somewhat difficult to diagnose a retropharyngeal abscess. The next diagnostic study you need is _____.

14. The CT scan shows a large retropharyngeal node that is ring enhancing and has a central lucency. Appropriate antibiotic coverage for this child would include covering the following organisms: _____, _____, _____, and _____.

15. A 2-year-old child is brought by her mother for treatment of sinusitis. She has been ill for 2 days and has a low-grade fever. Thick gray mucus is streaming from both nostrils, and her ears are clear. You should _____ her mother and not prescribe _____.

Answers

1. RECURRENT TONSILLITIS, CHRONIC TONSILLITIS, OBSTRUCTIVE SLEEP APNEA, ASYMMETRIC TONSILS
2. ADENOIDECTOMY
3. FOREIGN BODY
4. ACUTE EPIGLOTTITIS
5. BAG AND MASK VENTILATION
6. CROUP
7. BRONCHOSCOPE
8. CYSTIC HYGROMA
9. THYROGLOSSAL DUCT CYST
10. CERVICAL ADENITIS
11. ATYPICAL TUBERCULOSIS
12. LATERAL NECK X-RAY
13. A CT SCAN
14. S. PNEUMONIAE, H. INFLUENZAE, S. AUREUS, ANAEROBE
15. REASSURE, ANTIBIOTICS

NOTES

NOTES

NOTES

NOTES

NOTES

NOTES

NOTES

NOTES